CREATIVE FOOD
EXPERIENCES
FOR CHILDREN

CREATIVE FOOD
EXPERIENCES
FOR CHILDREN

Mary T. Goodwin
Public Health Nutritionist

Gerry Pollen
Early Childhood and
Elementary School Teacher

Center for Science in the Public Interest, Washington, D.C.

Design: Cynthia Fowler
Photographs: Lauren Versel
ISBN: 0-89329-001-7

14th Printing   (1st Printing of Revised Edition) January, 1980

We Are Delighted To Dedicate This Book
To Our Children
Jonathan, Rachel and Micah Goodwin
Karen And Meryl Pollen

We suggest that this book be used as a resource book by or for

Preschools
Daycare Centers
Elementary Schools
Parent Education Classes
Recreation Departments
Summer Camps
Scout Groups
Children's Television Programs
Parents
Senior Citizens
Physically and Mentally Handicapped People

Acknowledgements

We wish to express our thanks to Frances Moore Lappé for granting us permission to use the nutrition charts and several recipes from her book, *Diet For A Small Planet*.

We also thank the Moosewood Restaurant and Julie Jordan for allowing us to use recipes from their books, *Moosewood Cookbook* and *Wings of Life*, respectively.

To Lynn Dennie, Nutritionist, we would like to say thank you for the fine assistance you gave us.

Our thanks to Michael Jacobson, Ph.D., and Sandra M. Kageyama, M.P.H., and Bonnie Liebman, M.S., of the Center for Science in the Public Interest and to Alice Abramson, Executive Director of the Montgomery County 4C Council for their valuable suggestions, comments and encouragement.

We express our gratitude to the secretaries who worked patiently with us.

Acknowledgments

Contents

Introduction

I hear and I forget; I see and I remember; I do and I understand.

—Chinese Proverb

Children are the future of any society. The foods children eat affect their growth, development, ability to learn, and general behavior. How children eat is equally important. The presentation of food in a comfortable, relaxed atmosphere together with love, care and eye appeal, can greatly affect the child's self image and view of others. Early experiences with food may lay the foundation for lifelong eating habits.

Children learn most effectively by being actively involved. Therefore, children both at home and at school should be encouraged to be interested in food and involved in the preparation of their food. Children like food and are curious about living and growing things. Through such activities as planting seeds, watching them grow, and then caring for the plants, children learn to respect life and begin to sense their relationship to the world around them.

Food can offer an adventure, a way of discovering the world. For the child food is a symbol of love and security. Creating something beautiful and good with food is indeed a rewarding experience for anyone. In order to help children make the right food choices, a wide variety of wholesome foods should be available. Many opportunities should be given to explore the raw materials which are the sources of food such as grains, legumes, vegetables, fruits, nuts, seeds, etc. Consider the fun and excitement in sprouting and growing wheat. The child feels the wheat on the stalk, grinds the wheat into flour, makes dough out of the flour, shapes the dough into bread, smells the aroma of freshly baked bread, hears the crackle of the crunchy crust and finally tastes the flavor of hot homemade bread which he or she has had a hand in creating.

Creative experiences with wholesome foods are more important for children today than they were thirty years ago. Many children eat foods which come in boxes, packages, bags, bottles and vending machines and have been designed to be eaten on the run. Carefully prepared food invites us to come and to savor at the "welcome table". Misleading advertising glamourizes poor eating habits and encourages children to eat junk foods which may undermine their health.

Formulated, fabricated, fake foods (the 4Fs) are displacing wholesome foods in the diet. To protect children from food abuse, legislation is needed to control the production, sale and the accompanying advertising of these foods.

Children have to be educated to make good food selections. Food habits which build good health are not acquired naturally; they must be learned.

Children need to know how to take care of their bodies. They should know that their body parts are built during childhood and that wholesome food continually helps to maintain and repair their body tissues. The food which children eat is converted into body structure for growth and effective functioning throughout life.

Every child should be given the opportunity to learn about foods. They should know why foods differ and why it is necessary to eat many different kinds of food in order to grow to their genetic potential. When children help in the preparation of their own food, they are strengthening their self images and learning independence. A program for children which includes many food experiences is fun, informative and very valuable to them.

I. WHAT DOES THE CHILD LEARN FROM CREATIVE FOOD EXPERIENCES

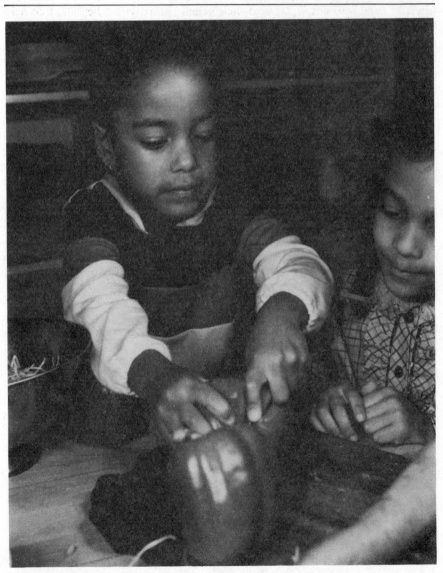

Learning
Experiences
Through Food

An Awareness of Nutrition

Young children will recognize the beneficial effects of eating wholesome foods through the study of nutrition and the vital role it plays in one's life. Children enjoy active play and they want to be healthy. Proper foods give them the energy they need to run and jump, to grow up, to be strong and active.

Emotional and Social Development

From birth, food is a symbol of love and security. Food comforts. Food nourishes. Food is an excellent vehicle for human communication. Love is expressed through serving food with care and delight. Sharing food and communication go hand in hand.

Food preparation can give the feeling that our efforts count. The success in creating something good to eat improves one's self image and self-confidence. Learning the skills necessary for cooking helps one to develop a sense of independence.

Through food we can discover that in some ways people are alike and in some ways people are different. People have different tastes. Joe liked the coconut as soon as he tasted it. Mary didn't like it.

Language Skills

There are many opportunities for children to learn new concepts as they prepare and eat food. When working with children, use the correct term for the food, the equipment or the process; *dissolve* powdered milk in water, *squeeze* oranges, *melt* butter, *pop* corn, *boil* water, *freeze* ice cream, *beat* eggs, *knead* dough, *peel* an apple, notice the *bitter* taste, etc.

Science

Early childhood is a good time to begin the study of the origin of food and growing things. How does a plant grow? What does a plant need to grow, where does it grow, when does it grow? What is an egg? Why does it hatch?

How does food make us grow and develop? What effect does food have on how we feel, look, and behave? When we are hungry, we get restless and irritated. The preparation of food also teaches us the value of making mistakes. If our results are not as the recipe described, we must solve the problem of why.

Mathematics

Buying, preparing and serving food calls for the development of a sense of quantity and measurement. Money, recipe measurements and timing, the dividing of portions, and the setting of the table all involve mathematics.

Art

Food can awaken the artist or the creative genius in everyone. Consider the satisfaction of making a beautiful loaf of bread. Colors and shapes may be learned through food. Apples are red or yellow or green. Pumpkins are orange and spinach is green. Grapefruit are spheres and are made up of sections. A carrot slice is the shape of a circle and milk cartons are rectangles. The colors, textures and shapes of food inspire creative expression.

Social Science

Through experiences with food, the child can become aware and appreciate the role of the family. He can come to understand that working together, sharing the tools and dividing the work benefits all. Children enjoy hearing about and seeing different foods from different countries. The differences in climate, soil and culture could be made to come alive through stories, pictures and projects. Children can discover much about their own families and ethnic background through food. Geography and transportation are major factors in determining the availability of foods.

Safety

The proper use of tools and ingredients for food preparation can be used to teach the principles of sanitation and safety.

Courtesy

Children should be guided to observe certain behavior while eating. Eating in an attractive and healthy manner by sitting straight in order to digest food, serving others before oneself, and taking a fair share of the food develops in the child a sense of self respect and respect for others. It also makes mealtime a more pleasant experience for everyone.

Potential Contribution of Food Experiences to Early Childhood Curriculum

All learning is through the senses. Food appeals to all senses, making it a powerful learning tool.

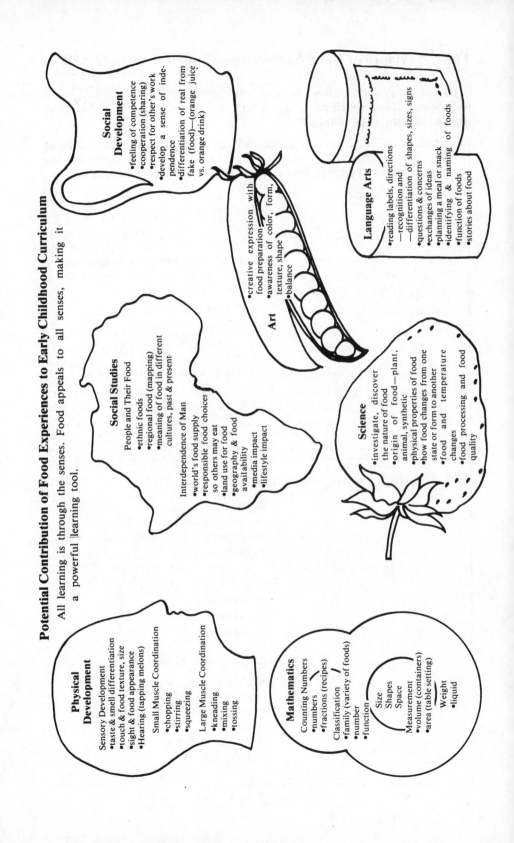

Social Development
- feeling of competence
- cooperation (sharing)
- respect for other's work
- develop a sense of independence
- differentiation of real from fake (food)—(orange juice vs. orange drink)

Language Arts
- reading labels, directions
  - recognition and
  - differentiation of shapes, sizes, signs
- questions & concerns
- exchanges of ideas
- planning a meal or snack
- identifying & naming of foods
- function of foods
- stories about food

Art
- creative expression with food preparation
- awareness of color, form, texture, shape
- balance

Social Studies

People and Their Food
- ethnic foods
- regional food (mapping)
- meaning of food in different cultures, past & present

Interdependence of Man
- world's food supply
- responsible food choices so others may eat
- land use for food
- geography & food availability
- media impact
- lifestyle impact

Science
- investigate, discover the nature of food
- origin of food—plant, animal, synthetic
- physical properties of food
- how food changes from one state or form to another
- food and temperature changes
- food processing and food quality

Physical Development

Sensory Development
- taste & smell differentiation
- touch & food texture, size
- sight & food appearance
- Hearing (tapping melons)

Small Muscle Coordination
- chopping
- stirring
- squeezing

Large Muscle Coordination
- kneading
- mixing
- tossing

Mathematics

Counting Numbers
- numbers
- fractions (recipes)

Classification
- family (variety of foods)
- number
- function

Measurement
- Size
- Shapes
- Space
- volume (containers)
- area (table setting)
- Weight
- liquid

The Importance of Good Nutrition and Food for Young Children

One of the greatest gifts we can give our children is good health and social well being. Good nutrition is the most important single factor for good health and optimal development.

FOOD EFFECTS

Physical Development

- growth
- development
- learning
- behavior

Children are building their bodies for life.

Social Development

- formation of eating habits
- take responsibility for food choices
- develop awareness of taking responsibility for personal health
- feel good about self

FOOD SERVICE

Model for Good Nutrition

- well balanced meals
- nutritious snacks
- using local and regional foods
- ethnic foods

Develop Skills

- food buying
- food preparation
- food service

Socialization at Mealtime

- feel good about self
- respect rights of others
- learn to relate across generations
- share—cooperate
- celebrations

A Brief
Perspective on
Food Education

Food and nutrition education is effective, fascinating and gratifying if taught in the context of the life situation and cultural backgrounds from which children come. Not only is the familiar being used as a point of departure. It is also a means of significantly enriching the lives of children by using food education to take them deep into positive aspects of their lives and culture. This builds a good self-image—an essential ingredient for effective learning of any kind. In addition, the uniqueness of each person is respected, at a time when many children feel faceless and forgotten. For the creative educator marvelous adventures are awaiting exploration. Some important tools for this expedition are knowledge of and responsiveness to each child's qualities and needs, a deep respect for each child and his/her uniqueness and efforts. The following outline is a guide on which to base the food and nutrition education program. It may be used as a beginning, a means, or an end. It is a sumptuous recipe for a delicious program to educate children to be their very best selves.

Food and the Child: Areas for Development

1. A good self-image through:
   a) knowledge to make wise decisions about food choices;
   b) skill to select quality foods and power to be an expert shopper;
   c) skill to prepare simple, nutritious meals promoting a sense of self-reliance;
   d) feeling competent to acquire these survival skills and able to use them.

2. An appreciation of being a healthy person is enhanced by:
   a) knowledge of how food promotes growth and development and nourishes the body throughout the life cycle;
   b) awareness of how to reduce the risk for diet-related illness and conditions.

3. Enjoyment of sensory development and experiences through:
   a) awareness of the sights, sounds, smell, feel and taste appeal of good food;
   b) food experiences providing subtle sensory refinement;

c) making use of sensory experience and pleasures for the development of good eating habits.

4. Appreciation of ethnicity through:
   a) recognition of one's uniqueness from personal history, roots, and their influences on food behavior;
   b) affirmation of self;
   c) recognition of and respect for the uniqueness of others;
   d) cultural sharing, and insights into other cultures.

5. Development of creativity as an expression of self, through:
   a) experimentation with the colors, forms, textures, smell and tastes of food;
   b) expressing oneself (myths, magic and mirth) through the art of baking;
   c) development of imaginative dishes, meals, ways of eating under current individual lifestyle constraints.

Food, the Child and the Community: Areas for Exploration

1. Promotion of socialization through:
   a) savoring the process of obtaining, preparing and serving food;

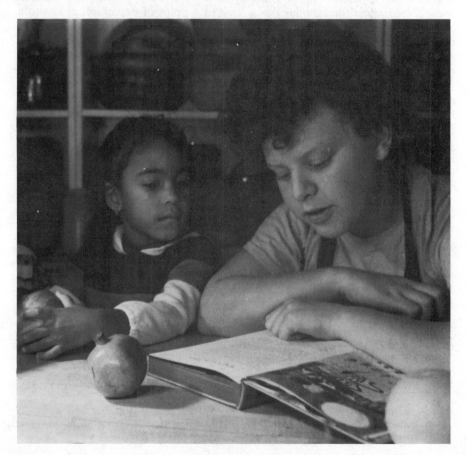

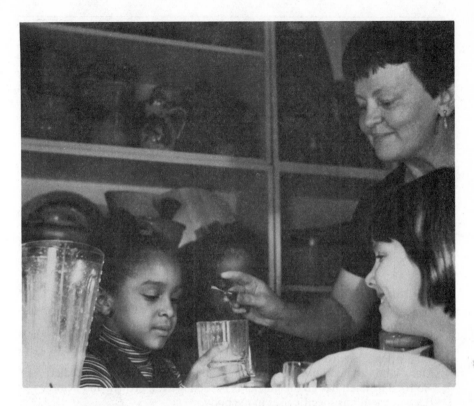

   b) food sharing increasing social participation;
   c) participation in rituals, traditions, festivals, and celebration around food evoke feeling of warmth, comfort, belonging and joy;
   d) recognition of the rhythms of life and death.

2. Enhancement of cross-generational relationships through passing of food skills from generation to generation promotes belonging, sharing, caring, and learning, and gives a perspective on family history.

3. Encouragement of regional awareness through:
   a) regional foods that put us in touch with our surroundings;
   b) pride in resources, when close to the source;
   c) respect for land that produces food;
   d) awareness of the rhythms of nature—food is our most direct contact with nature.

4. Promotion of sound ecology through:
   a) effective, and efficient, use of local land to provide higher quality, fresher, tastier, nutritious food;
   b) conservation of energy in transportation and storage;
   c) reduced pollution.

5. Develop an awareness of social responsibility through:
   a) eating patterns based on need, not greed;
   b) concern for others by encouraging conservation, cooperation, and sharing.

Basic Nutrition
Information

1. Nutrition is the food you eat and how the body uses it.
   We eat food to live, to grow, to keep healthy and well, and to get energy for work and play.

2. Food is made up of different nutrients needed for growth and health.
   All nutrients needed by the body are available through food.
   Many kinds and combinations of food can lead to a well-balanced diet.
   No food by itself has all the nutrients needed for full growth and health.
   Each nutrient has specific uses in the body.
   Most nutrients do their best work in the body when teamed with other nutrients.
   Some foods provide little nutritional value.
   Eating too much of some foods promotes disease.

3. All people throughout life have need for the same nutrients, but in varying amounts.
   The amount of nutrients needed are influenced by age, sex, size, activities and state of health.
   Suggestions for the kinds and amounts of food needed are made by trained scientists.

4. The way food is handled influences the amount of nutrients in food, its safety, appearance and taste.
   Handling means everything that happens to food while it is being grown, processed, stored and prepared for eating. For example, when vegetables are overcooked the nutrients are reduced.

A Brief Guide to Basic Nutrition Information

Nutrient requirements are dependent upon the body's need for 1) energy, 2) growth and development, 3) regulation and maintenance of bodily functions, and 4) the ability of the body to use nutrients.

The body needs: 1) water 2) energy (from carbohydrate, fat, or protein) 3) protein 4) essential fatty acids and fat soluble vitamins 5) water soluble vitamins, and 6) mineral elements.

Key Nutrient	Function	Deficiency	Sources	Comments
Carbohydrates (CHO) Simple (sugar) Complex (starch) Should supply 55-60% or more of energy (calories)	Provides energy.	Weight loss, fatigue, lowered resistance to infection.	Grains, cereals, breads, potatoes, corn, legumes, fruits, small amounts in vegetables.	% of calories from CHO in the American diet should be increased. Minimally processed foods contain a higher nutrient density along with energy—whole grains and fresh fruits and vegetables are best.
Fiber-Dietary Cellulose Hemicellulose Lignin Pectin	Promotes healthy bowel function, may help prevent colon cancer and control obesity and diabetes.	Diverticulosis, constipation, hemorrhoids.	Whole grain products (wheat berries, yellow cornmeal, whole barley, rye, oats) wheat bran, legumes, vegetables and fruits.	Whole grains with their full fiber content are best. Fiber is low in the U.S. diet.
Lipids Should supply 25-30% or less of energy.	Supplies large amounts of energy in a small amount of food. Promotes healthy skin by supplying essential fatty acids, helps body absorb vitamins A, D, E, K.	Dry, rough, itching skin. Poor growth. Unknown in the U.S.	Vegetable oils, meats, butter, cheese, egg yolk, nuts, milk, cream.	Calories from fat should be decreased. Excess dietary fat is a factor in heart disease and possibly some forms of cancer.
Protein Should supply 10-15% of energy.	Builds and repairs all tissue in the body. Helps form antibodies. Supplies energy.	Growth failure, lowered resistance to infection. Virtually unknown in the U.S.	Meat, fish, poultry, eggs, cheese, milk, yogurt, dried beans and peas, peanut butter, nuts.	Plant proteins may be eaten in combination for cheaper and lower fat protein sources.

A Quick Rundown on Vitamins and Minerals

Vitamins can be divided into two categories: water soluble and fat soluble. Fat soluble vitamins are stored in body tissues and can build up to toxic levels. Water soluble vitamins are excreted when taken in excessive amounts and are therefore less dangerous. Extremely high doses may overtax the body's capacity to excrete the excess, however, and damage may result. In general, the safest way to get enough vitamins is to eat a variety of wholesome foods.

Key Nutrient	Function	Deficiency*	Sources	Comments
Fat Soluble Vitamins VITAMIN A	Helps keep skin smooth. Helps keep mucous membranes firm and resistant to infection. Necessary for proper vision.	Night blindness. Lowered resistance to infection. Dry, rough, itching skin.	Liver, egg yolk, fruits, dark green vegetables, whole milk, vitamin A fortified skim milk, margarine, butter.	Laxatives decrease absorption. Substances made from vitamin A, called retinoids, are being tested as cancer preventing agents. These chemicals are different from vitamin A. Excessive amounts of the vitamin can be toxic and should not be taken without a doctor's supervision.
VITAMIN D	Helps the body absorb calcium and phosphorus.	Rickets, osteomalacia. Faulty bone growth.	Fish liver oil, fortified milk, sunshine converts substances in the body to vitamin D.	Excessive amounts may be toxic, possibly causing kidney damage and abnormal calcium metabolism.
VITAMIN E	Acts as an antioxidant, protecting fats in body tissues from deterioration.	Drastic deficiency not apt to occur, except in severe malabsorption or premature infants.	Green, leafy vegetables, wheat germ, oils (except coconut oil), nuts, liver.	Freezer storage lowers vitamin E content of fried food. Health claims for large supplements as yet unsubstantiated. More than 200 IU (20 times the RDA) reported to cause nausea and intestinal distress.

*Deficiencies of most vitamins are rare in the U.S. except in severely malnourished individuals. In most cases, symptoms of deficiency disappear when moderate amounts of the vitamin are consumed.

Key Nutrient	Function	Deficiency	Sources	Comments
VITAMIN K	Maintains blood-clotting factors.	Tendency to bleed excessively.	Dark green, leafy vegetables, soybean oil, egg yolk, liver.	Prolonged antibiotic and anticoagulant therapy can cause deficiencies. Can be synthesized in the intestine so body not dependent on a dietary source.
Water Soluble Vitamins VITAMIN B-1 THIAMIN	Helps release energy from food.	Beri-beri (characterized by numbness or tingling of toes and feet, paralysis of legs, atrophy of leg muscles). Sensitivity to noise and pain.	Wheat germ, nuts, pork, peas, whole grain and enriched bread and cereal, dried beans, meat, fish.	
VITAMIN B-2 RIBOFLAVIN	Helps the cells use oxygen. Helps keep eyes, skin, hair healthy.	Cracks at corners of mouth (cheilosis). Eye irritation. Dermatitis.	Milk, cheese, liver, chicken, legumes, whole wheat and enriched bread and cereals, dark green leafy vegetables.	Easily destroyed by light if in solution (as in milk).
VITAMIN B-3 NIACIN	Helps keep the nervous system, skin, digestive tract healthy. Enables the cells to use other nutrients.	Pellagra. Weakness, poor appetite, scaly dermatitis, mental confusion.	Peanut butter, fish, meat, poultry, greens, breads and cereals, sesame seeds, soybeans.	
VITAMIN B-6 Pyridoxine	Helps the body use and make protein.	Anemia. Mental disturbances. Dermatitis.	Wheat germ, whole wheat grains and cereals, eggs, bananas, legumes, organ meats, seeds, fish, meat, greens.	Pregnancy, oral contraceptives, and excessive use of alcohol substantially increase need.

Water Soluble Vitamins Cont'd.

	Function	Deficiency	Sources	Comments
PANTOTHENIC ACID	Helps release energy from food.	Nervous disorders, decreased antibody formation.	Eggs, milk, legumes, liver, wheat bran, wheat germ, peanuts, peas, poultry, corn, asparagus, broccoli, sweet potato, kale, fish.	Deficiency unlikely.
VITAMIN B-12 COBALAMIN	Assists in manufacturing blood, production of sheaths surrounding nerves.	Anemia. Irreversible neurological damage.	Liver, kidney, meat, milk, cheese, oysters, fish, yogurt (not in plant foods)	Vegetarians eating no eggs or milk should take vitamin supplement.
FOLACIN FOLIC ACID	Involved in blood formation, cell reproduction and other biological functions.	Anemia.	Yeast, whole grains, legumes, cowpeas, lentils, navy and kidney beans, liver, asparagus, corn, broccoli, greens.	Pregnancy, oral contraceptives and excessive use of alcohol increase need.
VITAMIN C	Needed for synthesis of collagen, the cementing material that holds body cells together. Helps body resist infection. Strengthens blood vessels. Helps heal wounds and broken bones. Keeps gums healthy.	Scurvy characterized by listlessness, fleeting pain in legs and joints, small hemorrhages under the skin, bleeding gums. Lowered resistance to disease.	Kale, brussel sprouts, strawberries, broccoli, collards, mustard greens, green pepper, canteloupe, citrus fruit.	Easily destroyed by heat, exposure to air and by addition of baking soda when cooking vegetables. Health claims for large supplements as yet unsubstantiated.
BIOTIN	Synthesis of fatty acids. Helps release energy from glucose.	Deficiency unlikely.	Eggs, liver, pork, chicken, salmon, sardines, cauliflower, cowpeas, green peas.	Deficiencies produced by eating large amounts of raw egg whites (cooking destroys the anti-biotin factor).

A Quick Rundown on Vitamins and Minerals Continued

Key Nutrient	Function	Deficiency	Sources	Comments
Minerals CALCIUM	Bone and tooth formation. Blood clotting. Muscle contraction and relaxation.	Rickets. Poor growth.	Milk, cheese, sesame seeds, egg yolk, meat, legumes, whole grains, nuts, green leafy vegetables, mustard greens and collards, tofu.	High protein intake raises requirement.
PHOSPHORUS	Bone formation.	Poor growth (dietary deficiency not likely to exist)	Milk, cheese, meat, egg yolk, whole grains, legumes, nuts.	May be excessive in U.S. diet. A high phosphorus-to-calcium ratio may cause bone deterioration.
IRON	Serves as a constituent of heme, a part of the hemoglobin molecule.	Anemia, fatigue, listlessness.	Liver, meat, eggs, soybeans, molasses, green leafy vegetables, dried fruits.	Anemia is the most common deficiency disease.
IODINE	Component of thyroxin, a hormone which regulates the rate that the body uses energy.	Simple goiter.	Sea food, iodized salt, processed foods.	May be excessive in U.S. diet due to considerable amounts in processed foods.
MAGNESIUM	Regulates cardiac, skeletal muscle, and nervous tissue function.	Tetany. Convulsions. Muscle dysfunction.	Whole grains, pumpkin seeds, nuts, eggs, fish, green vegetables.	Alcoholics have increased need. Deficiency symptoms rarely occur—only in malabsorption, or alcoholism.

Mineral	Function	Deficiency Symptoms	Sources	Comments
SODIUM	Maintains fluid balance in body (osmotic pressure).	Weakness, fainting.	Table salt, processed food, monosodium glutamate, baking soda, sodium phosphate.	U.S. diet is too high in sodium. May contribute to the development of hypertension.
POTASSIUM	Necessary for muscle contraction and regular heart rhythm.	Muscular weakness and paralysis.	Fresh fish, green beans, red beans, milk, grapefruit, oranges, bananas, tomatoes, spinach.	May help prevent hypertension.
CHROMIUM	Helps in metabolism of glucose.	Impaired glucose tolerance.	Meats, whole grain bread and cereal, brewer's yeast.	Growing concern that U.S. diet may be deficient in chromium.
ZINC	Promotes growth and wound healing.	Impaired growth. Defective healing. Impaired sense of taste. Loss of appetite.	Oysters, peas, whole grain cereals, liver, oatmeal, beef, clams, corn, peanut butter, milk.	Growing concern that U.S. diet may be deficient in zinc.
COPPER	Promotes iron absorption and utilization, helps maintain blood vessels, nervous system, and bones.	Anemia, bone fragility, nervous disorder.	Nuts, liver, raisins, dried beans and peas, shellfish.	Some concern that U.S. diet may be deficient in copper.

II. A GUIDE TO INVOLVING CHILDREN IN FOOD EXPERIENCES

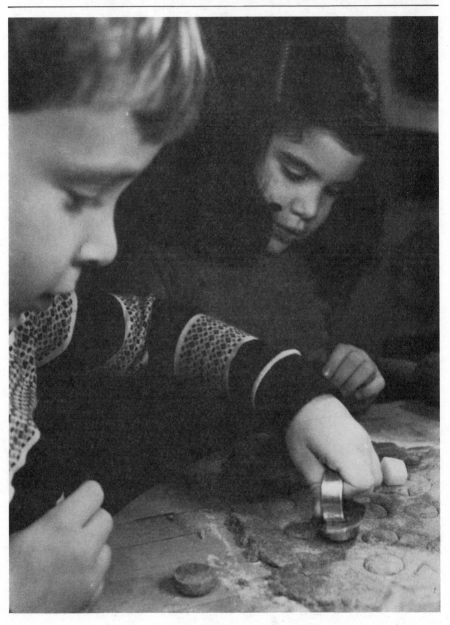

Cooking Is Easy When We Learn the Correct and Safe Way

Planning for the Cooking Experience

1. At first, cooking projects should have few steps such as taking peas out of a pod, making gelatin pudding, popping corn or making cranberry sauce in order to give the children the experience of working with food. The careful washing and preparing of vegetables and fruits is another single activity.
2. Gradually, the experience could become more complex by incorporating more steps.
3. Always be receptive to the children's suggestions if they are within reason as to what they would like to make.
4. Be alert to the many ideas for food preparation which arise spontaneously out of other activities and experiences.

Preparation for Cooking

1. Post a chart of the recipe where it can be easily seen. This chart should include pictures of the utensils needed along with pictures illustrating the measurement of ingredients, such as a drawing of two teaspoons for 2 teaspoons. See illustration below:

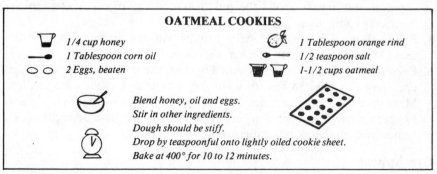

OATMEAL COOKIES

1/4 cup honey
1 Tablespoon corn oil
2 Eggs, beaten

1 Tablespoon orange rind
1/2 teaspoon salt
1-1/2 cups oatmeal

Blend honey, oil and eggs.
Stir in other ingredients.
Dough should be stiff.
Drop by teaspoonful onto lightly oiled cookie sheet.
Bake at 400° for 10 to 12 minutes.

2. Gather the group and explain the necessity of washing hands and putting on aprons.

3. Cooking projects are easily managed if the group is no larger than 5 or 6.
4. Make sure work surface is clean and point this out to children, explaining why.
5. Go over recipe and all directions carefully with children before starting.
6. Have a tray of utensils ready with enough utensils available to keep the project moving. More than one child at a time might have a turn, if possible.
7. Have another tray of ingredients ready.
8. Have a clean sponge and a bowl of water available for quick clean-up.
9. Show the children how to use the utensils properly and supervise their use.

Safety
1. Help children become aware of sharp knives, graters, parers.
2. Keep all potentially dangerous utensils away from young children. Under very careful supervision, they might be able to use a grater or a plastic knife.
3. As the opportunity arises during cooking, point out the dangers of very hot water, the danger of burnable objects too near the stove, the importance of turning off appliances after using them.
4. Make sure all pot handles are turned toward the back of the stove and tell the children why; make sure handles are turned away from the edge of the table.
5. Show the children how pot holders are used to avoid burns.
6. Young children should not use the stove top or oven and should stay away from the stove.

While Cooking With the Children
1. Everyone should have a chance to see, smell, feel and possibly taste ingredients before they are combined.
2. Help children observe and talk about contrast, color, texture, size and shape.
3. Help children observe and talk about what happens when ingredients are combined, such as the effects of temperature on food. Express in words that water is a *liquid;* when it boils, it changes into a water *vapor* called steam; when it freezes, it changes into a *solid* called ice.
4. Use complete sentences and the correct words for all actions, objects and concepts, but always accept the child's unique way of expressing ideas or describing something.
5. Follow through on projects. After helping with the preparation, everyone should have a chance to taste what was made.
6. Encourage all those who participated to share the responsibility of cleaning up. Show the children how to wash the utensils and sponge the surfaces. Make sure all utensils are clean before putting them away. Even if a spot has been missed, recognize the effort of little hands. Improvement in skill comes from guidance, not criticism.

Eye Appeal
1. Since the eye eats first, the food should be appealing to look at as well as to eat.

Glossary

Bake—Cook in oven.

Baste—Moisten food while it is cooking (as meat while roasting) by spooning liquid or fat over it.

Batter—Mixture of flour and liquid, or in combination with other ingredients, thin enough to pour. Used to coat foods for frying.

Beat—Mix vigorously over and over with a spoon or fork, or round and round with a beater.

Blanch—Dip in and out of boiling water to loosen the skins of fruits or nuts.

Blend—Mix thoroughly two or more ingredients until smooth.

Boil—Cook in steaming liquid in which bubbles break on surface.

Bread—Coat with flour, eggs and crumbs.

Broil—Cook directly under heating unit in range or over hot coals.

Chill—Allow to become thoroughly cold.

Chop—Cut into pieces with knife or chopper.

Coat—Cover with thin film as flour, fine crumbs, icing, sugar or crushed nuts.

Cool—Let stand at room temperature until no longer warm.

Cream—Combine 2 or more ingredients by rubbing or beating items until they have lost their individual appearances.

Cube—Cut into 1/4-1/2 inch cubes.

Cut in—Mix fat into flour mixture with a pastry blender, a fork or two knives.

Dice—Cut into very small cubes.

Dot—Drop bits of butter or cheese here and there over food.

Dough—Mixture of flour and water in combination with other ingredients, thick enough to roll, knead, or drop off a spoon.

Drain—Pour off liquid.

Dredge—Coat with flour or crumbs.

Drizzle—Pour gently from a spoon.

Dust—Sprinkle lightly with flour or sugar.

Flake—Break lightly into small pieces.

Flour—Dust greased pans with flour until well coated on bottom and sides. Shake out extra flour.

Fold—Mix gently, bringing rubber scraper down through mixture, across bottom, up and over top until blended.

Frost—Cover with icing.

Garnish—Decorate with pieces of colorful food such as parsley, pimento, cherries or lemon.

Grate—Rub against grater to cut into small pieces.

Grease—Spread bottom and sides of pan with shortening.

Grind—Cut or crush in a food grinder.

Knead—Work dough with your hands by repeating a folding-back, pressing-forward and turning motion.

Marinate—Cover beans or meat with a well seasoned sauce and let stand to flavor.

Melt—Heat until liquid.

Mince—Chop or cut into tiny pieces.

Mix—Combine ingredients, as by stirring.

Pan-Fry—Cook in small amount of fat in skillet.

Pare—Cut off outside skin, as from apple or potato.

Peel—Pull off outer skin, as from orange or banana.

Pit—Remove pits or seeds from fruit.

Roast—Cook by dry heat.

Roll-out—Flatten and spread with a rolling pin.

Scallop—Bake in a sauce with crumbs and/or grated cheese on top.

Score—Make series of shallow cuts on surface of a food.

Shred—Cut into very thin strips.

Sift—Put through flour sifter or fine sieve.

Simmer—Cook in liquid almost to boiling but not hot enough to bubble.

Slice—Cut a thin, flat piece of large food mass, such as meat loaf or roast.

Soak—Immerse in liquid for a time.

Steam—Cook in the steam produced by the boiling of water or other liquid.

Stir—Mix round and round with spoon.

Toast—Brown by direct heat.

Toss—Mix lightly.

Whip—Beat with rotary egg beater or electric mixer to add air.

Food Preparation
and Language Arts*

Language skills, both listening and speaking, are developed through food preparation by *using* the correct term for the food, the utensils and the equipment and for the process taking place. This list is a reference list for the teacher and may be expanded.

How many of these terms and concepts have you used? How and when do you use them?

Action Words

combine	spread	squeeze	pour
scrape	stuff	peel	dissolve
beat	sprinkle	pit	cool
pop	butter	stem	measure
crack	skin	pare	warm
ice	sizzle	core	chill
whip	bubble	let rise	yields
refrigerate	stir	grease	drop
grate	heat	soften	bite
grind	sift	compress	cut
boil	chop	knead	chip
simmer	dice	halve	add
bake	slice	quarter	melt
broil	strain	toast	press
divide	steam	roll	preheat
brown	freeze	shape	chew
cool	melt	mix	swallow
digest	coat	smell	drizzle
nut	cover	scrape	fold
toss	dredge	crack	dip

*This material has been adapted from a handout prepared for Delaware-Maryland Head Start written by Sandra Horowitz.

Temperature

hot	cold	cool	warm
degrees	heat	preheat	boiling
chill	lukewarm	frozen	steaming

Time

instant	overnight	next day	minute
gradually	alternately	second	quickly

Size

large	small	little	tiny
huge	miniature	bite-size	chunks

Shape

round	square	circle	oblong
cube	rectangle	oval	fluted

Quantity

degrees	cupful	a dash	more
package	quart	enough	ounce
pint	square	pinch	teaspoon
a few	less	double	whole
dozen	long	slice	cup
tablespoon	some	approximate	half
both	pound	short	bunch

Ingredients

ginger	nuts	baking powder	juices
parsley	nut meats	yeast	ade
sage	coconut	cream of tartar	evaporated milk
rosemary	cheeses	grains	powdered milk
thyme	beans	legumes	sour milk
salt	rind	lentils	whole milk
cinnamon	stem	grated peel	skimmed milk
cornstarch	leaves	seeds	homogenized milk
brown sugar	stalk	fruits	pasteurized milk
honey	gelatin	vegetables	eggs
molasses	vanilla	meats	oil
shortening	whole wheat flour	fish	peanut butter
margarine	white flour	poultry	baking soda
butter	rye flour	rolled oats	wheat germ

Flavor

tart	bland	mild	mellow
bitter	sweet	tangy	sour
spicy	salty	blend	

Texture

mealy	wet	stringy	creamy
smooth	stiff	dry	firm
tender	hard	compressed	crunchy
crisp	lumpy	mushy	moist
rough	tough	soft	granular
sticky			

Mixtures

batter	dough	sauce	gel

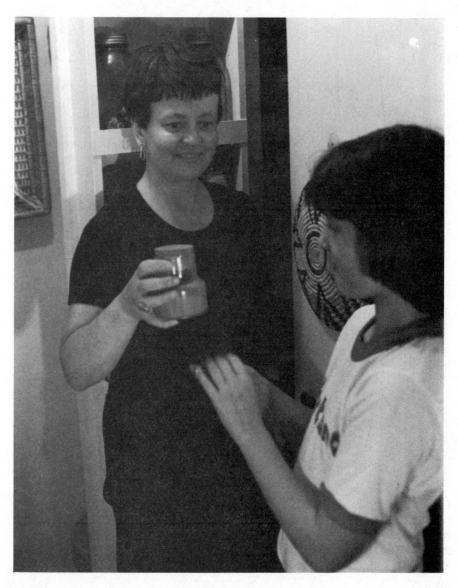

Utensils We Use

For Preparation

knife	apple corer	grater	can opener
vegetable parer	kitchen scissors	fruit juicer	cutting board
vegetable brush	colander	wire strainer	food grinder
			food mill

For Measuring

graduated measuring cups	straight-edged spatula	rubber scraper	liquid measuring cup
sifters		measuring spoons	

For Mixing

wooden spoon	knife and fork
pastry blender	rubber scraper
mixing bowls	rotary egg beater
wire whisk	

For Top of Range Cooking

heavy skillets	pancake griddle
double boiler	pancake turner
saucepans	

For Baking

13-inch oblong pan	wire rack	two 8- or 9-inch layer pans	rolling pin with cover
9-inch pie pan	cooky cutters	muffin pan	casserole dish
pot holders	cooky sheet	8-inch pan	
9-inch loaf pan	wide spatula	cake tester	
	biscuit cutters		

How Do We Measure?

1. Children can learn the importance of measuring specific amounts of food ingredients when cooking and baking.
2. Before you begin baking with the children, demonstrate the difference between unsifted and sifted flour:
   a. Allow a child (keep the groups small) to pour the unsifted flour into a measuring cup and level off.
   b. *Transfer* the flour into another container.
   c. Have another child sift this same flour into the same measuring cup.
   d. Talk with the children about what happened. What did they observe?
3. As you cook or bake with the children and the need arises, demonstrate and then allow the children to:
   a. *Pack* butter or margarine into a measuring cup.
   b. *Pack* bread or chopped celery, onions or nuts into a measuring cup until level with the top.
   c. *Pack* brown sugar into measuring cup by pressing down with the back of a spoon. Sugar should hold its shape when turned out of the cup.
   d. *Level* off the butter or margarine with a spatula or table knife.
   e. *Level* all teaspoon and tablespoon measurements.
   f. *Pour* the desired amount of liquid (milk, water, oil, etc.) into a measuring cup which is standing on a table. Have the children bend down to look at the mark at eye level to be sure the amount is right.
4. Remind children not to pour over the mixing bowl in case of pouring too much.
5. Use nesting-type measuring cups as well as graduated measuring pitchers.
6. If you are doing the measuring, talk about what you are doing.
7. If the children are measuring, suggest that they measure carefully.

In order to expose the children to a different method of measuring amounts during food preparation, try weighing the ingredients. (See Granola recipe #2 in Recipes section, page 247.)

III. FUN WITH FOOD LEARNING ACTIVITIES

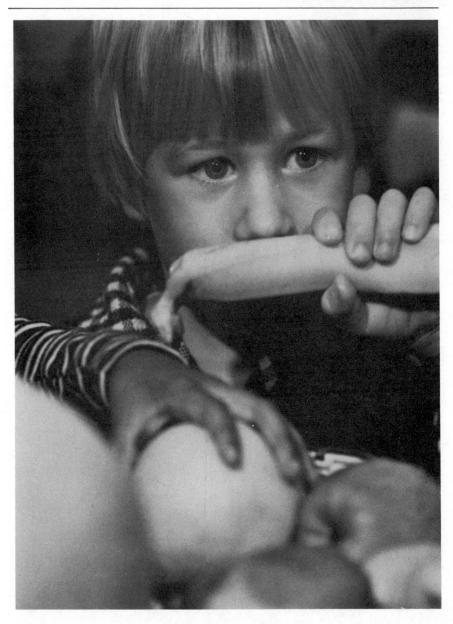

Fun With
Food Learning
Activities

Teacher's Note:

1. The purpose of this section is to introduce children to and encourage the consumption of a variety of wholesome foods.

2. Please don't let your own food prejudices interfere with the selection and presentation of new and/or different foods.

3. It is important that adults working with children be notified of any food allergies that their children may have.

4. Explain to children why it is necessary to chew popcorn and nuts thoroughly. Chewing food well helps to prevent choking.

5. If cost is a factor, concentrate on the less expensive foods such as powdered milk, whole grain cereals, and low cost seasonal fruits and vegetables.

6. Depending on the activity and the ages of the children, divide the class into small groups and rotate the activities.

7. Use your judgment as to how many items to include in any one lesson involving comparisons. For example, lesson #2 under milk may be broken down into more than one activity or some of the milk forms could be eliminated. Availability of the milk forms, cost, and group size may also limit your selection.

8. Since children learn through sensorial experiences, emphasize feeling, smelling, observing and listening to the sounds foods make during preparation, cooking and eating.

9. To make this section come alive and to make it fun:
    a. Plan a theme for the day such as Hi Ho the Dairy Oh!
    b. Use the theme as a focus for the food experience.

    c. Enrich these experiences with music, songs, dance, art, dramatic plays, stories, games, celebrations, parades and field trips.

    d. Post a recipe chart with illustrations for each food project.

A few enrichment suggestions are made with each of the lessons. There are many other possibilities which we hope you will experiment with and develop.

10. When working with this activity section, refer to the following sections:

    a. A Guide to Involving Children in Food Experiences (II)

    b. Suggested Activities for Expanding the School Food and Nutrition Curriculum (IV)

    c. Sources and Resources (V)

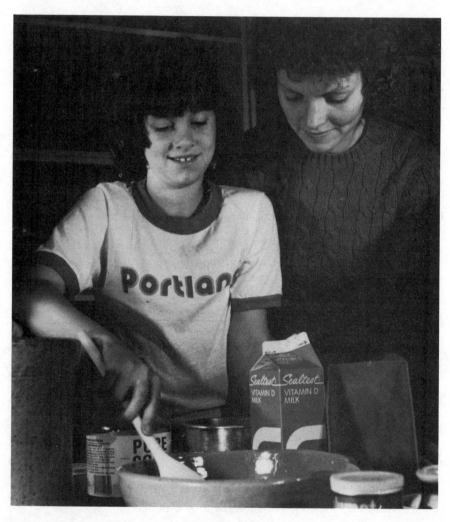

You Are Magnificent!

Part 1

Objective:

The children will experience through their senses that their bodies are good and should be respected.

Materials:

Songs for singing
Music for dancing
Posters and pictures of food

Procedure:

1. Encourage the children to explore, experience and appreciate that their bodies are great. What can you do with your body?

   a. Our eyes give us the pleasure of seeing beautiful things. What are some of the beautiful things around you?

   b. Our ears are for hearing. Now listen in silence for two minutes. Report all the sounds you heard when you were still. Walk outside and listen to the birds, wind in the trees, traffic sounds, etc.

   c. Our nose is for smelling. Smell the spices. Which is your favorite?

   d. Our tongue is for tasting. What are your favorite foods?

   e. Our teeth are for chewing. Do you chew food slowly and enjoy it?

   f. Our hands are for touching. How many different textures are around you? Feel them and describe them (Table—smooth, rug—soft, etc.) Our hands are for clapping.

   g. Our feet are for walking, dancing, running.

2. What other things can you do with your body?
   Sing and make beautiful music.
   Do a dance that involves the whole body in creative expression. Make up a song and dance to celebrate the senses.

We should love our bodies and give them what is good for them. Our bodies do wonderful things because they are us.

Eating good food is one way of saying we care about ourselves. The food we eat becomes us.

Is your grandmother or grandfather living? Do you want to live to enjoy a long life?

3. Your body is you and you can do wonderful things. Name some of them. You show love and respect for your body by eating the food your body needs to grow, develop and function properly.

The nutrients in food build and repair the tissues of the body. Some tissues are hard like the bones and teeth. Some are soft like muscles and skin. Some are fluid such as blood, saliva and tears. All these tissues are made up of the food we eat, the water we drink and the air we breathe.

For shiny hair and healthy eyes, your body needs dark leafy green and deep yellow vegetables. Name some.

For strong bones and healthy teeth, your body needs calcium supplied by milk and cheese. How much milk do you drink?

Your blood needs iron rich foods such as dark leafy green vegetables, meat, dried beans and peas, whole or enriched grains. Why do you need healthy blood?

To help protect your body from infections, you need vitamin C found in citrus fruit, tomatoes, cabbage, potatoes, and green vegetables. Which do you like best?

To regulate your body and keep it running well, you need fiber, vitamins and minerals. Whole grains, fruits, and vegetables do a fine job.

For growth and body repair, protein foods supply the needed materials. Fish, eggs, dried peas, beans, meat, nuts, seeds are excellent protein foods.

4. Your body is for life. Build it well and take care of it. It is you!

People both young and old need good food to keep them healthy.

Maybe the children could talk to an older person about which foods they ate which kept them in good health. Or, perhaps they ate too much sugar which caused tooth decay or didn't exercise their gums enough with fruits and vegetables.

Impress upon the children that now is the time to build healthy bodies and establish good eating habits. Eating habits are learned. Children are not born with them.

5. Do you have pets at home or in class? Do you feed them food to make them grow and keep them healthy?

Taking care of pets and finding out what their food needs are would be an excellent class experiment.

Teacher's Note:

Two excellent books to use with these activities are *Faces* and *Bodies* by Barbara Brenner. See Resource Section for details.

You Are Magnificent!

Part 2

Objective:

The children will see that each child is an individual with his own size, shape, weight and height. The food each child eats affects these characteristics.

Materials:

Tape measure for each child
Felt, 5' x 8'' for each child
Dowels about 7'' long for each child
Scale for weighing
Felt pens
A variety of pieces of colored felt
Cord or string
Camera—instant
Height and weight table
Baby pictures of each child (if available)

Procedure:

1. Discuss with the children that each person is different physically and in other ways. Genetics and the food we eat and how our body uses it determines:

   Size and height—tall or short
   A good diet is very important for a child to reach his or her genetic potential.

   Shape and weight—thin or fat
   What is ideal for the individual: Too little food may result in undersize and thinness. Too much food may result in obesity. The proper amount of food will result in the proper weight.

   Appearance—Bright eyes and clear skin are indicators of a good diet.

   Energy—Calories in food give us energy. Other nutrients help the body use the energy. Children with poor diets may be tired and listless. Children with well-balanced diets are likely to have lots of energy for work and play. Children grow at different rates and at different ages.

2. Which foods could you eat to make your body even more beautiful than it is?
   The children could write or draw a book on the foods their body needs.

3. What foods should you avoid or eat once in a while to protect your body?
   Sugar causes tooth decay. What foods contain sugar?
   Foods high in saturated fat should be limited, especially if someone in your family has heart disease. What are some of these foods?

   Very salty foods should not be eaten too often, especially if someone in your family has high blood pressure. What foods are these?

   Foods debased by excessive amounts of artificial coloring and artificial flavoring, refined flour, and excessive sugar are potentially harmful to our health. Can you name some of these?

4. Make your own tree of life. If an instant camera is available, take pictures of each child and use them for his or her tree of life.

   Paste a 60 inch tape measure on a piece of felt about 8 inches wide and at least 60 inches long, with the beginning of the tape at the bottom of the felt. Fold the top of the felt over the dowel, glue the felt down, making a pocket to enclose the dowel. Put the cord or string on each end and hang. Have each child choose and cut out a symbol for the top, such as a flower, a smiling face, a photograph, etc. Paste the symbol at the top. The measure is used for the tree of life. Decorate the sides with leaves or fruit or other nutritious foods.

5. Measure each child on his or her own tree hanging and mark the child's height. Weigh each child on the scale and mark it on the child's tree.

6. Compare the child's baby photograph with his or her present size. Discuss how food plays a role in his or her growth and development from birth to the present time.

7. Post baby pictures and play a game matching baby pictures with the right child.

8. It would be a wonderful experience for the children to invite a mother and baby to visit and talk about how everyone was a baby once. Have the children compare themselves to the baby in size and behavior. Explore what role food plays in this development.

Teacher's Note:

Here is another appropriate activity for *You Are Magnificent:*

1. Pair the children. Have one child lie down on the sheet of paper while the partner traces the child's outline. This may also be done by tracing a shadow on a wall using the sun or an opaque projector.

2. Have each child fill in how she or he sees himself or herself.

3. Point out that some are tall, some are short, some are slender, some are well rounded, some are in-between. No two are exactly alike; each person is special.

4. Point out differences that may result from food and how it is eaten. The food that is eaten affects growth and development.

5. Nutrition is concerned with the future of the individual.

Your
Food Shield

Objective:

The children will discover the meaning of food in their lives and their own unique food habits.

Materials:

Pictures of shields with coats of arms.
A large piece of newsprint for each child.
A set of crayons, felt pens or paints for each child.

Procedure:

1. Discuss with the children:

   What is a shield?

   - Something that protects, a broad piece of armor
   - It has a coat of arms on it which contains an insignia reflecting some unique characteristics of the bearer

   What is a food shield?

   - Something to symbolize the protection of the health and social well being of the bearer.
   - It has a coat of arms on it which reflects each individual's unique food preferences.

2. Have the children draw with the felt pen or crayon a large outline of their favorite food to use as the shield.

3. Ask each child to use a felt pen or crayon to divide his/her shield into six parts.

4. Select six of the following categories and ask each child to draw one of each for the six spaces on the food shield.

   a) Favorite food a parent prepares for the child
   b) Foods fished, hunted or gathered—wild foods, garden foods, or from the supermarket (chosen by the child)
   c) Favorite ethnic food, or regional food

d) Foods he/she eats when happy
e) Foods he/she eats when sad
f) Foods the child feels his/her body needs
g) Favorite food for celebrations

5. Guide the children in a discussion of their food shield, why these foods are important to them, and how they protect and comfort them.

Teacher's Note:

This activity is a good way to put the children in touch with their feelings about food. Food nourishes, protects and provides security. The coat of arms depicts the child's unique food habits.

This activity lends itself well to learning projects related to biblical times, middle ages, etc., through which the children can discover how and why shields were used.

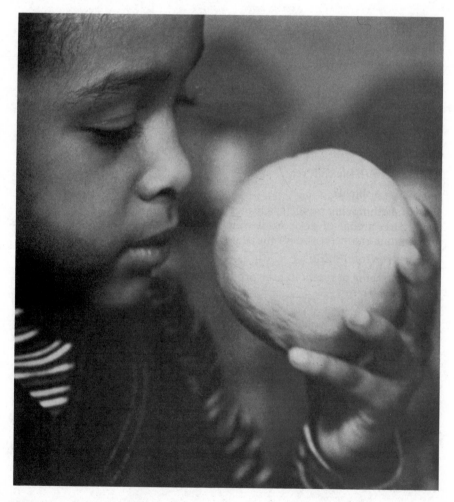

Come to
Your Senses

Objective:

To explore the sights, sounds, smell, touch and taste appeal of food.

Introduction:

Through our senses we are in touch with ourselves and the world around us. The quality and depth of our involvement depends on our sensory development. All learning is through our senses. Food has the potential to be one of our richest learning experiences because it appeals to all the senses. We expand or limit, enjoy or deprive ourselves through the quality of our sensory experiences. Today all too many of us are culturally depriving ourselves and our children by limiting our food experiences to taste for sugar, fat and salt. The challenge is to liberate your senses in the marvelous world of food. The object of the following activities is to savor the subtle sights, sounds, smells, touch and tastes of foods. Allow time for sensory absorption. A great adventure for all ages to encourage eating more fruits, vegetables and grains.

ACTIVITY I: SIGHTS—The food rainbow—see and remember.

1. Fill a farm basket with as many colorful fresh fruit and vegetables available. (Participants may bring in a fresh fruit or vegetable for this activity.) Here are some ideas:

   Primary colors: Red—apples, tomatoes, strawberries, watermelons
   Yellow—banana, lemon, yellow string beans, squash
   Blue—blueberries, blue plums, blue grapes

   Secondary colors: Purple—eggplant, bermuda onions, red cabbage
   Orange—oranges, tangerines, persimmons, pumpkins
   Green—peas in a pod, avocados, celery, broccoli

2. Encourage participants to examine the various shades and tints of color within each fruit and vegetable. Some fruits like apples come in a variety of colors. Compare the inside and outside colors of foods. Suggest participants note how colors change with cooking. Emphasize the visual delight of color.

ACTIVITY II: SIZES AND SHAPES—The minute to the monumental.

1. Take a trip to a supermarket or fruit and vegetable stand—identify the many shapes and sizes, from tiny red currants to huge watermelons; from stalks of rhubarb to egg-shaped mangoes; from soft curly endive to crisp flowerets of broccoli. Consider the seemingly endless variety.
2. Compare the insides of fruits and vegetables, whether layered (artichokes, brussel sprouts, cabbages, onions), hollow (peppers), firm (eggplant, potato, apples), juicy (strawberries, oranges, melons), or seeded (pea pods, pomegranate, tomatoes).
3. Collect samples of dried beans and peas; green and yellow split peas; red and brown lentils; garbanzo, fava, aduki, kidney, pinto, soy, mung and black turtle beans. Compare subtle differences in shapes and sizes.

ACTIVITY III: SOUNDS—Listen and hear.

Ask participants to describe food sounds or tape these sounds and ask participants to identify them from the tape.

1. Gathering—apples dropped into a basket, slosh of milk in a coconut.
2. Preparation—popping of corn or cranberries, sizzling of fish under a broiler, bubbling of soup, simmering of stew, chopping of celery, slicing of bread, spreading of peanut butter, squishing of garlic through a press, beating batter for bread, grating of orange rind, kneading of dough, cracking of eggs, squeezing of a lemon, shucking of corn, crushing of nuts, crackle of crusty bread.
3. Eating—crunching nuts, chewing raisins, biting into an apple, swallowing orange juice, chomping on a raw carrot, squishing a cherry tomato.

ACTIVITY IV: SMELLS

1. Put a variety of herbs and spices in separate small containers. Some suggestions—Herbs: fresh or dried a) parsley, b) sage, c) rosemary, d) thyme, e) basil, f) oregano, g) dill, h) tarragon, i) spearmint, j) anise; Spices: a) cinnamon, b) cloves, c) ginger, d) nutmeg, e) cardamon, f) coriander, g) chili powder, h) paprika, i) turmeric.

   Place a number on each for identification. Ask participants to sniff and write the name of each on a piece of paper.
2. Obtain whole roots, seeds, barks or leaves from which herb or spices are made. See whether they can be identified whole and if not, what must be done to elicit their aroma.
3. Discuss favorable food smells—freshly baked bread, stuffed chicken roasting in the oven, tomato sauce simmering on the stove, peeling of oranges, chestnuts roasting on an open fire, apples baking, granola browning.
4. Discuss or visit places that smell of foods. (Open markets, ethnic restaurants, community festivals, neighborhood bakeries, herb and spice or tea shops). Have participants sniff their way through a supermarket and identify the smells, or drive or walk by a fast food restaurant and sniff. Or suggest they sniff their way around a farm.

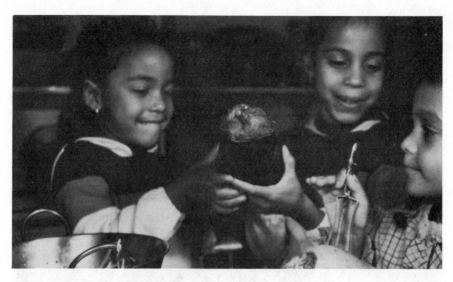

ACTIVITY V: FINGER FOOD FEEL AND MOUTH FOOD FEEL

1. Put fruits or vegetables into a paper bag one at a time. Have participants put one hand in the bag and feel the food carefully, discovering its textures and shapes. Ask them to identify the food. The following are some suggestions:

fuzzy—peach
waxy—apple
firm—carrot
soft—persimmon
hard—winter squash
hairy—kiwi
bumpy—cauliflower

sleek—eggplant
prickly—pear
seedy—raspberries
light—bell pepper
heavy—pomegranate
sticky—dates
moist—strawberries

2. Wash the fruits and vegetables and cut them in pieces the size of finger foods. Have each participant eat a piece slowly and describe the mouth feel.

ACTIVITY VI: TASTE OF LIFE—A time to feast.

1. Collect a wide range of raw fruits and vegetables. Here are some suggestions:

sweet—strawberries, pineapple, mango
sour—cherries, lime, rhubarb
sweet and sour—kiwi, kumquat (massage before eating to blend flavors)
pungent—onions, garlic
bitter—radish
strong—turnip, brussel sprouts

mellow—cantaloupe
creamy—persimmon
tart—plum
snippy—watercress
sharp—mustard greens
spicy—apple
tangy—raspberries
bland—mushrooms, cucumbers

2. Have participants take a sample of as many as desired and eat each slowly, savoring the flavor. Discuss familiar tastes, new tastes, favorite tastes.

Note:

These are great classroom activities for young and old. If budget is limited, select a few characteristic foods. Learning to enjoy new foods is a little like learning a new language. Some learn quickly and others slowly. Activities may be repeated using different forms of the same basic foods to increase sensory awareness and pleasure.

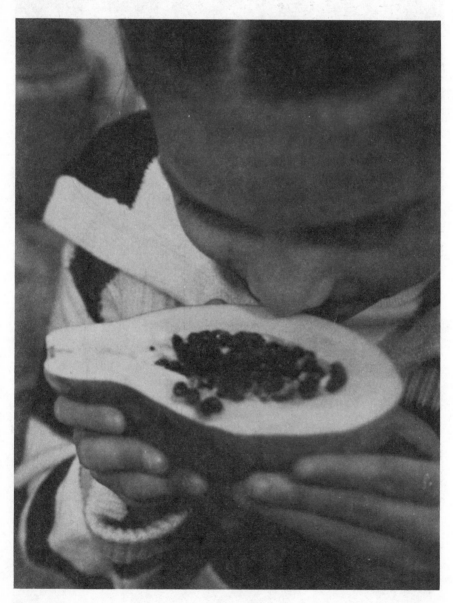

Vegetables

Vegetable #1:

See How Vegetables Grow

Objective:

The children will plant and care for a vegetable seed to discover how vegetables are grown.

Materials:

Pot of parsley
Pitcher of water
Green felt pen
Construction paper, white
  and brown

Bowl
Pot of earth, or individual cups
  with earth for each child
Seeds (beans, radish, corn,
  parsley—these grow
  relatively quickly)

Procedure:

1. Show the children the pot of parsley.
2. Cut off a sprig for each child.
3. Discuss the bright green color, the curly shape, how long the seed may take to grow into a plant for food.
4. What does the parsley seed need to grow?

   It needs food from the seed and the soil, water from the rain, light from the sun. See: *Growing Things in the Classroom,* Section IV.

5. Wash the parsley well. Have everyone taste the parsley. Does the parsley taste good?

6. Ask the children, "What are your favorite vegetables?" "Would you like to plant a seed and grow your own vegetables?"

7. Let each child select the seed he or she wishes to plant. Push the seed down and cover it with earth. Water the seeds and put them in the sun.

8. Make a calendar for four weeks with the white construction paper and green felt pen. Cut out small brown pots for 10-14 squares. Have children take turns pasting a brown pot on the calendar each day while waiting for the seeds to sprout. When the first green shoot appears, paste on a green leaf. Vegetables grow very s-l-o-w-l-y.

9. Activities while waiting for the vegetables:

    Have children make pictures of how their plants are growing.

    Try sprouting mung beans. Mung bean sprouts are good to eat as they are, or try them in a salad or sandwich. See *Vegetable Seeds Are Very Good Indeed!* Section III.

    Visit a neighbor's garden and see how beans grow. See *Growing Things in the Classroom,* Section IV.

    Have the children look at large seeds and sprouts under a magnifier. Point out how the germ of the seed grows and how the energy for growth comes from the starchy part of the seed. Soy and lima beans are especially good for this.

Vegetable # 2:

Underground Vegetables

Objective:

The children will investigate some vegetables which grow underground.

Materials:

Radishes	Scraper
Beets	Paring Knife
Carrots (with tops if possible)	Large paper bag
Potatoes (white or sweet)	Pictures of other root
Turnips	vegetables growing
Onions	Cutting board

Procedures:

1. Vegetables are plants.
    We eat many parts of the plant.
    The part of the plant that grows underground is the root.
    Do you know what underground vegetables are called?
        Root vegetables. Tuberous (potato) and fleshy (carrot) roots are the kind you eat.
    Do other plants have roots?
    What are roots for? Through the roots, the plants are furnished with food and water from the soil.

2. Vegetables, like potatoes, are planted in the soil.
   The plants grow until the potatoes are ready to harvest.
   A big machine digs up the potatoes.
   The potatoes are put in bags and trucked off to the market.
   Where do you get your vegetables?

3. Point out that most root vegetables have a skin to protect them.
   Some skins such as carrot skin may be eaten, but onions should be peeled because the skin has a bitter taste.

4. Pass around the root vegetables; discuss the color and texture of the skin (smooth, silky, bumpy, rough).
   Which vegetables are good to eat raw or cooked?

5. Plant radish seeds in the classroom. They should be ready to eat in 2 or 3 weeks.
   Radish roses can be made by cutting off the stem end, leaving a bit of the stem. Cut thin petals from stem to root end around radish. Place in ice water to open. This would make a nice garnish in a salad.

6. Play a guessing game.
   Put the vegetables in a bag.
   Close the bag, leaving enough room for a small hand to slip in and out.
   Ask each child in turn to put his or her hand in the bag, pick a vegetable, name it, and pull it out to see if the naming is correct.

7. Have the children wash, scrape, or grate a vegetable. If a carrot is prepared, make carrot sticks. Carrot curls can be made by slicing scraped, raw carrots lengthwise with a slicer into paper-thin slices. Roll up and fasten with a toothpick. Place in ice water to curl carrots.

8. Why are root vegetables good to eat?
   They give us energy. Deep yellow vegetables such as sweet potatoes, carrots and rutabaga are rich in vitamin A. Vitamin A is important for healthy eyes. Vegetables contain fiber and minerals for maintaining healthy bodies. Vegetables which are eaten raw stimulate gums, clean the teeth and promote good dental health.

Read:

The Great Big Enormous Turnip, A. Tolstoy
The Carrot Seed, R. Krauss

Teacher's Note:

For additional lessons, try boiling well-scrubbed potatoes. Let the children mash them, add butter or margarine and salt. Serve the potatoes for snack or lunch. Compare hard raw potatoes with soft cooked potatoes. Eat hot potatoes with cold sour cream.

The term *deep yellow* vegetables does not include vegetables such as corn, which would not be a high source of vitamin A.

Some Vegetable Stems Are Good To Eat

Objective:

The children will investigate which vegetables have stems that are good to eat.

Materials:

Mushrooms	Celery	Asparagus
Rhubarb	Carrots	Cheese
Peanut butter	Raisins (optional)	Nuts (optional)

Poster on versatile vegetables from the Green Giant Company Home Services. (Remove brand name label for classroom use.)

Toothpicks

Procedure:

1. Discuss stems.
   What is a stem?
   Which stems do children know (flower, boat, glass, torso of a person)?
   How would you dramatize these ideas?

2. Where is the stem on a vegetable?
   The stem is the part between the roots and the leaves.

3. What are stems for?
   The stem carries the food from the root to all parts of the plant.
   The stem supports the plant as the trunk supports the tree.
   See *Learning About Science*, Section IV: the celery and colored water experiment.

4. Which stems to we eat?
   Celery, asparagus and mushrooms.

5. What can we do with stems like celery?
   Wash and cut them into sticks, about 2" long.
   Stuff them with peanut butter. Make celery curls by slitting both ends in narrow strips, almost to the center. Place in ice water to curl ends.
   Make a celery wagon. Cut 2" long sticks of celery. Attach round slices of carrots with toothpicks for wheels. Fill the wagon with nuts, raisins, cheese.

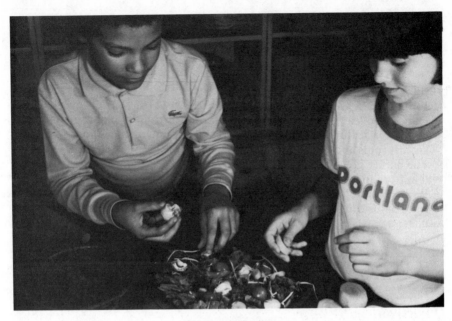

Vegetable #4:

Dark Green Leaves For Us To Eat

Objective:

The children will examine and taste plant leaves which are good to eat.

Materials:

Lettuce	Salad dressing
Spinach	Colander
Cabbage	Large bowl
Kale	Small covered saucepan
Parsley	Paring knife
Collard	

Procedure:

1. Animals such as deer eat leaves. Why does the giraffe have a long neck?
   The long neck makes it possible for the giraffe to reach the leaves at the
   top of the trees.
   Do you know other animals that munch on leaves?
   Where do we find the leaves on plants?
   What sort of stems do plants with leaves have?
   Some plants with leaves have roots we can eat; which ones are these?
   People eat leaves, too.
   Do you know what leaves we eat? Cabbage, lettuce, brussel sprouts,
   spinach and beet greens.
   Encourage each child to taste each kind. Discuss color (light or dark
   green), texture (crisp, limp, firm, thick), size of leaf (small or large),
   taste (mild, bitter, sweet).

2. Discuss which greens are usually eaten raw, cooked, or either way. Discuss which way the children like them best.

3. Have the children wash and tear the lettuce, spinach and parsley into bite-size pieces (save some for cooking). Toss with salad dressing and serve for snack or lunch. Do the (leaves) greens taste differently in a salad?

4. Why are dark green leafy vegetables good for us?
   Dark green leafy vegetables are rich in iron for healthy blood, rich in vitamin A for healthy eyes, hair and skin, and rich in vitamin C to help protect against colds and infection.
   The darker green the vegetables, the higher in food value. These also contain fiber and other minerals.
   While vegetables such as lettuce are not dark green and, therefore, not a rich source of vitamin A, they do provide a source of fiber and bulk to the diet.

Vegetable #5:

Please Eat These Flowers

Objective:

The children will examine flowers that are vegetables. They will discuss flowers that are good to eat.

Materials:

Cauliflower	Paring knife
Broccoli	Saucepan
Water	Bowl
Salt	Pitcher
Butter or margarine	Colander
Cutting board	

Procedure:

Talk about flowers:

1. Bees like flowers because some flowers have nectar.
   The bee uses the nectar to make honey.
   Do you know some of the flowers bees like? Clover, orange blossoms, blackberry blossoms, apple blossoms.

2. Can you name some flowers people like to eat?
   Cauliflower, broccoli, nasturtiums, violets.
   Which flowers are vegetables?
   Try making dandelion tea.

3. Pass around the cauliflower and broccoli.
   Discuss the shape of the cauliflower or broccoli.
   Discuss how it feels, looks, smells.
   Talk about its color and texture—rough, smooth, hard or soft.

4. Put the vegetables in a colander and wash well under running water.

5. Separate the plant into individual flowers or florets. Ask the children to taste them. How do they taste?

Make broccoli hearts by removing one-quarter inch of the outer part of the thick lower stem.

6. Cook the remainder of the vegetables in a small amount of boiling water. Drain and season cooked vegetables. Save the liquid to make soup.

7. Taste and compare the texture, color and flavor of the raw and cooked vegetables. Save some of the raw vegetables to help the children with the comparison.

8. What has the heat done to the vegetables? It has softened the cellulose. Which way do you like your vegetables best? Raw or cooked? Do you like a sauce on your vegetables?

Teacher's Note:
A cauliflower is a compact mass of underdeveloped flowers.

Vegetable #6:

Fruits That Are Vegetables

Objective:
The children will see, taste, feel and talk about fruits that are vegetables or fruit-vegetables.

Materials:

Eggplant	Basket for vegetables
Peppers	Cutting board
Tomatoes	Paring knife
Squash	Bowl
Okra	Pitcher
Cucumber	Vegetable brush

Procedure:
1. What is a fruit?
   Fruits are juicy and fleshy.
   Fruits have beautiful colors and wonderful shapes.
   Some fruits are soft and others hard and crunchy.
   The pulp of the fruit is the tissue which encloses the seed or seeds.
   We call some vegetables fruit-vegetables because they are the fruit of the plant.
   Do you remember the other parts of the plant?

2. Which vegetable has your favorite color?
   How does each vegetable feel? Waxy, spongy, firm, crisp, limp, soft, hard, prickly, slippery, heavy, light, rough, smooth.
   Talk about the shapes of these vegetables: funny, round, oblong.
   Can you guess how many seeds are inside?
   Are the seeds big or small?
   Are the seeds in the middle of the fruit or all over the inside?

3. Wash the vegetables well and cut each open to look, see and feel.
   Are there empty spaces inside or is the fruit filled with pulp?

4. Taste how good vegetable-fruits are.

5. What can you do with these vegetables?
   You can eat them raw as snacks or in salads. You can cook them by boiling, baking or steaming. You can eat them with sauces or in casseroles.

Teacher's Note:

Check the recipe section for easy ways to serve vegetables in the classroom. If facilities permit, try Squash Soup or Chicken Gumbo made with okra, eggplant and parmesan. Serve for lunch. Children should taste and enjoy a wide variety of foods in many forms. Okra was brought to America from Africa. It is used in the South for thick soups and gumbos.

Don't forget to plant seeds. See *Growing Things in the Classroom,* Section IV.

Have the children dramatize how different vegetables look and feel.

Vegetable #7:

Vegetable Seeds Are Very Good Indeed!

Objective:

The children will experiment with vegetable seeds by cracking, chewing, popping, planting, sprouting and drying.

Materials:

Peas in pods	Bowls (3)
Corn for popping	Mason jars
Green string beans (fresh)	Salt
Soy or mung beans (for sprouting)	Cookie sheet
Peanuts in shell (raw)	Popcorn maker

Procedure:

1. What is the seed of a plant?
   The seed is the part of the plant from which a new plant (new life) will sprout.

2. Seeds are very nutritious.
   They contain protein for growth, vitamins and minerals for healthy bodies, and energy for work and play.

3. Vegetable seeds are good to eat.
   Let us name some: peas, corn, beans, peanuts.

4. What can we do with a vegetable seed?
   Wash the *sweet pea* pods. Open and remove the sweet peas. Cook them.
   Wash the *string beans* and remove the stems. Open a few and look at the seeds. Eat them raw or cooked.
   Roast raw nuts on a cookie sheet. Open a roasted *peanut shell* and eat the nut. Plant *raw* peanuts outside and watch them grow. Roast at 325 °F. for 20 minutes.
   Corn is for shucking and/or popping. Try shucking when corn is in season, cook and feast. Chew popcorn well!!
   Popping *corn* is fun for a party.

Mung beans and *soybeans* sprout easily. Put some soy or mung beans in a large jar with water. Soak overnight, drain off the water and put in a dark, dry, warm place (closet). Rinse with cool water twice a day. *Observe changes daily*—changes in size, hardness or softness, color, new shoots. The sprouts should be ready to eat in a few days. Try them in salads or sandwiches.

5. If you have a garden, harvest your *green beans* or buy fresh whole string beans. Dry some for stews and soups in the winter time. Mountain people dry them and call them *"leather breeches"*. Fill a long needle with a long, strong thread. Push the needle through the center of the bean, pushing the beans together at the end of the thread. Hang in the warm air, but away from direct sunlight. Observe changes occurring day by day. Let them remain hanging until the beans become dry. Store in a bag until ready to use. Try them in soups, stews, and casseroles. In Appalachia, some mountain folk preserve them this way. Why do we preserve food?

Vegetable #8:

Vegetable Garden Soup

Objective:

The children will observe the changes that occur when vegetables are cooked.

Materials:

Root—onions, carrots   Salt
Stem—celery   Pepper
Leaves—parsley   Beef bouillon
Flower—cauliflower   Paring knife
Fruit—tomatoes   Colander
Seed—peas   Soup kettle
Others, if desired

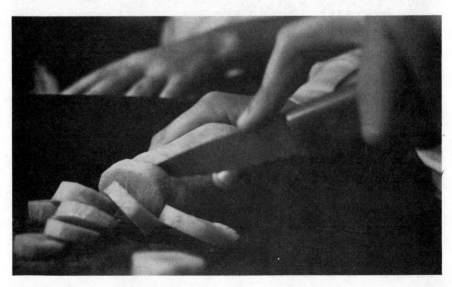

Procedure:

1. Read *Stone Soup* by Marcia Brown.
2. Take a trip to a garden or supermarket to select vegetables for soup, or have each child bring a vegetable from home.
3. Have the children wash the vegetables well and prepare them for the soup.
   The vegetables should be about the same size so they will cook in about the same time.
   Heat about 2 quarts of water in the soup kettle until hot. *Be very careful.*
   Remove the pan from the heat.
   Very carefully, have one child at a time drop his or her vegetables into the pot.
   Cook until the vegetables are tender.
   Season with salt and pepper.
   Serve for a snack or lunch.
4. Discuss the effect of heat on the vegetables. How does cooking change the texture, flavor, color and aroma of each vegetable?
   Give the children the opportunity to taste and compare the raw and cooked vegetables.

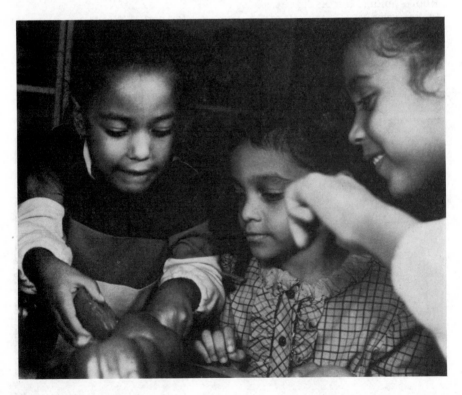

Fruits

Fruit #1:

What Can We Do With An Apple?

Objective:

The children will investigate many characteristics about apples.

Materials:

Medium-size fruit basket
Paring knife
Water
Bowl
Cutting board
Scale (optional)

Small, medium and large apples:
    Golden-Yellow Delicious
    Red-Stayman
    Green-Rhode Island Greening
    Speckled—McIntosh

Apple Products:

Applesauce
Apple juice
Apple cider
Apple vinegar

Apple jelly
Baked apple
Dried apple
Apple butter

Procedure:

1. Wash apples well. Why? This removes dirt, bacteria (germs), and pesticides. Put apples in the basket.

2. Getting to know all about apples.
   Pass the basket of apples around, asking each child to pick out an apple.
   What *color* are the apples? Red, green, yellow, speckled.
   What *shape* are the apples? Round, pear shape.
   What *sizes* are the apples? Small, medium and large.
   Which apples are heavy; which apples are light; which are the same?

Why are apples *different sizes?* Genetics, soil, and climate.

How do apples *smell?* Sweet and sour.

How do apples *feel?* Hard, smooth and waxy.

How do apples *taste?* Sour or sweet, spicy or mild, tart or bland.

How do apples *sound* when we eat them? Quiet or loud, soft or crunchy, crisp.

What *covers* the apples? A skin called peel.

Does the peel taste different from the pulp inside?

Why does the apple have a peel?

What are other parts of the apple? Stem, blossom, core and seeds.

What *color* are apples *inside?* White or pale yellow.

Into what *shapes* and *sizes* can apples be cut? Halves, quarters, thirds, circles (with stars in the center), cubes, shreds.

Is the apple dry or juicy when cut?

What happens if a slice of apple is exposed to the air? It turns brown. Why? Refer to teacher's note.

What happens if a slice of apple is dipped in salted water or orange or lemon juice? It does not turn brown. Why?

3. Why are apples good to eat? They taste delicious, look good, feel good, give us energy, help keep our bodies in good condition, clean our teeth, and keep our gums in good condition. They contain some vitamin C and dietary fiber.

4. What can we make with apples? See, touch, smell and possibly taste the products made from apples:

applesauce	apple butter
apple juice	apple jelly
apple cider	dried apples
apple vinegar	baked apples
apple relish	

How do you like apples?

apple juice	apple pudding	apple cake
apple salad	applesauce	apple pie
apple crepes	apple cookies	apple crisp
apple omelet		

5. Where do apples come from?
Plant an apple seed and watch it grow.
> See *Learning About Science,* Section IV and *Growing Things in the Classroom,* Section IV.

In spring time, bring in apple blossoms and enjoy their beauty. Discuss how fruit is formed from the blossom. Observe color, aroma, shape, size.

6. How many different kinds of apples can you name?
Which apples are your favorites?

Filmstrip:

How Apples Grow—National Apple Institute, Washington, D.C. or prepare a graphic presentation of how apples grow—a flannel board works well for this.

Song:

"I Climbed Up The Apple Tree" from *Rooster Crows**

Field Trips:

to an orchard
a roadside stand
fruit section in supermarket
apple tree in someone's backyard

Teacher's Note:

Oxygen in the air reacts chemically with substances in fruits and vegetables (oxidation). This process changes the color and flavor and reduces the content of certain vitamins. Oxidation in fruits and vegetables can be prevented by dipping the fruit in vinegar (an acid) or salted water (about one-fourth teaspoon per cup of water) or in ascorbic acid found in orange or lemon juice.

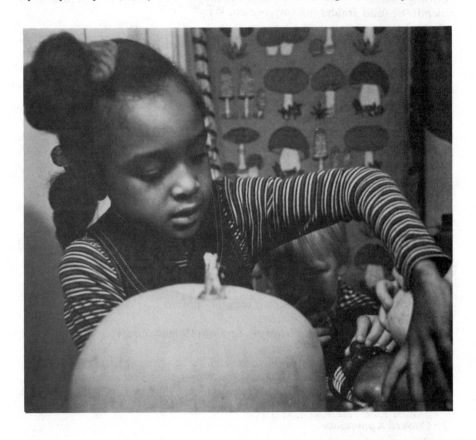

*Peter Miska and Maude Miska, McMillan Co., New York, 1945

Fruit #2:

Let Us Make Applesauce

Objective:

The children will observe the changes made by grinding apples to make raw applesauce.

The children will observe how heat changes apples by making cooked applesauce.

Materials:

Raw Applesauce

Paring Knife
Bowl
Pitcher
Cutting board
Blender or food grinder

3 apples
Water
Cups and spoons
1 teaspoon brown sugar
   or honey

Cooked Applesauce

Paring knife
Bowl
Pitcher
Cutting board
Sieve, strainer or food mill
3 apples

1 teaspoon brown sugar
   or honey
Saucepan
Wooden spoon
Cups and spoons

Procedure:

1. **Raw Applesauce**

   Wash 3 apples well.
   Pare if desired.
   Cut into medium-size pieces.
   Grind in food grinder or put a small amount of water in a blender and grind.
   Turn on blender and add a few pieces at a time.
   Taste applesauce.
   Add 1 teaspoon honey or brown sugar, if desired.
   What changes occurred?
      Consistency: solid whole apples to a soft, thick liquid.
      Color: white to light brown
      Taste: bland, mild, sweet or sour
      Smell: sweet or spicy
   What does the grinding do to the apples? It breaks down the cell walls (cellulose).

2. **Cooked Applesauce**

   Wash 3 apples well.
   Cut them into quarters.
   Place in a saucepan.
   Add just a little water.

70

Cook slowly until tender.

Strain or force through sieve or food mill.

Add 1 teaspoon of honey or brown sugar, if desired.

What changes occurred? See suggestion under raw applesauce.

What does heat do to the apples? Heat softens the fiber or cellulose. The cell walls collapse. The apple becomes soft and mushy.

3. If both methods are used for preparing applesauce, compare the color, consistency, texture and taste.

4. Try a little spice on applesauce like cinnamon, ginger cloves, nutmeg, all-spice. Does the spice change the flavor of the applesauce? Discuss.

Fruit #3:

Let Us Make Jackstraw Salad

Objective:

The children will combine apples with other foods.

Materials:

Bowls for vegetables	3 Carrots	Peanut butter
Paring knife	4 Large stalks celery	Cheese cubes
Cutting board	Salad dressing	2 Large green peppers
Serving spoons	Toothpicks	5 Large red apples
Plates for everyone	Forks for everyone	1 Head of lettuce

Procedure:

1. Wash carrots and celery well.
   Cut in thin sticks about 3 inches long.
   Cut celery and green peppers in thin slices.
   Cut apples in sticks, leaving the peel on ends.
   Combine.
   Toss with a small amount of salad dressing, if desired.
   Serve on lettuce—eat.

2. Put peanut butter on an apple wedge.
   Put a cube of cheese on a toothpick.
   Have a tasting party.

3. How do apples taste with other foods such as fruit, vegetables, peanut butter or cheese?

Teacher's Note:

Waldorf Salad is also a good recipe to use for a class project. Combine diced apple with raisins, nuts and chopped celery. Try orange sections, bananas, and grapes for variety. Moisten salads with salad dressing, squeezed lemon or yogurt, if preferred.

Fruit #4:

Where Do We Get Our Fruit?

Objective:
The class will discuss where we get our fruit.

Materials:

Peaches	Colander or strainer
Pineapple	Cutting board
Banana	Paring knife
Strawberries	Toothpicks
Blueberries	Globe or map

Pictures of fruit growing on trees, bushes, vines and plants.

Procedure:

1. Discuss how fruit grows on *trees* (apples, peaches, persimmons, oranges, etc.), *bushes* (blueberries, currants, gooseberries), *vines* (strawberries, pumpkins, melons) and *plants* (bananas grown in bunches).

2. How does the fruit come to us?
   Farmers grow the fruit.
   Workers or machines pick the fruit from the trees, plants, bushes or vines.
   The fruit is packed into boxes, baskets or crates.
   Trucks take the fruit to the grocery store.
   Some fruit comes to us from other countries by ship, train, truck or plane.

3. Where does fruit grow?
   Name the fruits that grow in your state.
   Ask the children if they grow fruit at home.
   Do they pick wild fruit such as berries anywhere.
   Is fruit available all year? Discuss which fruits we are able to buy fresh during spring, summer, fall and winter. Do prices of fresh fruits vary with season?
   Use the globe to discuss the countries from which we import fruit, like bananas from Central America where it is very warm all year.

4. During which seasons and climate does fruit grow best?

5. Fruit is good to eat just as nature grows it. What other ways can we buy fruit? Canned, frozen, dried.

6. Discuss size, shape, color inside and outside, texture and ripeness of the above fruits. Wash and prepare fruit for fruit kabobs. Serve as snacks or for lunch.

7. Take a trip to:
   a. an orchard—at blossom time when the green fruit is forming at harvest time
   b. cider factory
   c. outdoor market
   d. neighbor's garden with fruit trees or vines
   e. pumpkin patch

    f. take a walk to a wooded area and look for berries

    g. visit the Botanical Gardens

8. Look at a picture of an apple tree.

Ask: "Did you ever pick an apple from a tree?"

"How can you get them down from the top of the tree?"

"Where would you go to see an apple tree?"

Visit an apple orchard where the children can pick apples from the low branches of an apple tree, or visit a classmate's backyard where there is an apple tree.

Use the record, *Autumn* (Bowmar Catalogue*) and follow the section on picking apples from a tree. (Action song)

Tell the story, "Buttons and the Magic Apples" by W.L. Jenkins.**

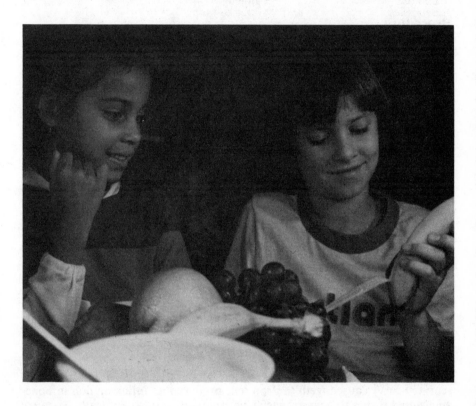

*Bowmar Catalogue, Glendale, California

**"Buttons and the Magic Apples," *Church Kindergarten Resource Book* by Josephine Newberry, John Knox Press, Richmond, Virginia, 1960

Fruit #5:

The Citrus Family

Objective:

The children will be introduced to similarities and differences in the citrus family.

Materials:

Orange	Kumquat (optional)
Tangerine	Quince (optional)
Lime	Grapefruit
Lemon	Tangelos

Procedure:

1. Compare members of citrus family.
   How are they similar?
   How are they different?

2. Wash well, cut open and compare.

3. Taste the different fruits and compare.

4. Why are citrus fruits important to our diet?

   Citrus fruits are important to our diet because they contain vitamin C.

   a. Vitamin C helps protect us against infections.
   b. Vitamin C is necessary to make the cementing material which holds our body cells together.
   c. Vitamin C helps heal wounds and broken bones.

5. Discuss Jacques Cartier, his crew and scurvy.*

6. Grow citrus fruit plants. —See page 155.

7. What are some of the other sources of vitamin C?

   Green vegetables such as collards, spinach, parsley, green pepper and kale; white and sweet potatoes.

8. Read: "Get Aboard the Good Ship Vitamin C", distributed by the Florida Citrus Commission, Lakeland, Florida.

Teacher's Note:

Many of those who died before the time of the Crusades probably died of scurvy. Scurvy caused teeth to drop out, produced an inflammation in bones and caused tissues to hemorrhage. This eventually resulted in death. Today a milder deficiency of vitamin C produces bleeding gums, sore bones and a tendency to bruise easily. During the 17th Century, it was discovered that lemons in the diet eliminated scurvy. Lemons and foods mentioned previously contain vitamin C, the only nutrient that can prevent scurvy.

---

*Cartier's expedition was forced to spend a winter near Montreal in 1535. He wrote in his log that he cured his dying men "almost overnight", simply by giving them a brew made from the needles of the pine tree. This was an Indian cure.

Fruit #6:

What Can We Do With An Orange?

Objective:

The children will examine oranges in comparison to orange juice and orange drinks.

Materials:

Navel oranges	Orange squeezer
Florida oranges	Frozen orange juice
Valencia oranges	Canned orange juice
Mandarin oranges	Tang
Tangerines	Hi 'C'
Cutting board	Orangeade
Paring knife	Small paper cups for everyone

Procedure:

1. See the section on apples—many of the same procedures can be repeated.

2. Pass the oranges around.

   Look at the skin, noting those which have thick skins and those with thin skins. (Navel oranges have a thick skin at the blossom end of the fruit.)

   Which orange is heavy?

   Which orange is light?

   Heavy ones have more juice.

   Which orange is large?

   Which orange is small?

3. Cut the oranges in half crosswise.

   Which one has seeds?

   Which one does not?

   Peel the orange; observe segments.

   Taste the orange.

   Squeeze juice from the orange.

   Taste the juice. What makes the juice different from the segments?

   Taste the different juices and drinks from the list above.

   Find out favorites and why?

Teacher's Note:

Oranges are high in vitamin C and also contain a modest amount of vitamin A. Orange juice—frozen, fresh or canned—is also very nutritious. Tang, Hi 'C', Kool-Aid and Orangeade are *synthetic*. Natural fruit juices come from fruit grown in an orchard. Synthetic drinks are basically chemical products made in a factory. Most contain unnecessary sugar, artificial coloring, flavoring, and preservatives which may be harmful to children. Natural fruit juice is good and wholesome and contains small amounts of many nutrients that are not added to the synthetic drinks.

75

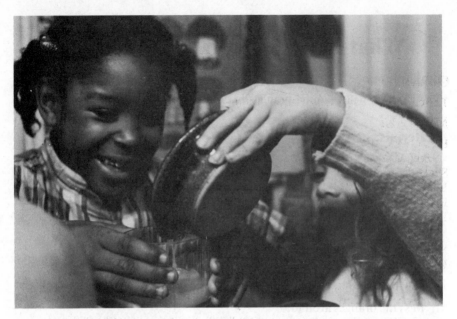

Fruit #7:

Let's Make An Orange Milk Shake

Objective:

The children will combine orange juice and milk to make a shake.

Materials:

Orange juice —1 cup   Ice —a few ice cubes
Powdered milk —1 ½ cups   Pitcher
Water —3 cups

Procedure:

1. Dissolve milk in water.

2. Add orange juice, mix well.

3. Add ice and serve.

4. Popsicles can be made by pouring the shake into popsicle containers and freezing.

Teacher's Note:

A small amount of milk added to the juice of an acid fruit such as orange, lemon, tomato, etc. will curdle the milk into curds. If a larger amount of milk is combined with the acid fruit juice, as in the shake above, no curdling occurs.

When milk curdles, the protein coagulates or clumps together. This can be caused by the acid in foods. When there is a high ratio of milk to acid, curdling is not likely to occur.

Try an experiment by adding a small amount of milk to a large amount of orange juice, such as 1 tablespoon of milk to 1 cup of orange juice.

Fruit #8:

Making Raisins

Objective:

The children will preserve fruit by removing the water from the fruit.

Materials:

Fresh, ripe, firm seedless Thompson grapes (enough for each child to have a few)

Scales

Large pan or bowl of water

Plastic-coated trays or paper plates

Pieces of clean cheesecloth, mosquito netting, or wire screen, large enough to cover the trays.

Glass container with tight-fitting lid

Procedure:

1. Weigh the grapes and record the weight. Handle the grapes carefully as they bruise easily. Save a few for comparison later.

   Place the grapes in the container of water and wash them thoroughly.

   Lift the grapes from the water and blot them with a towel.

   Remove the grapes from the stem and spread one layer of grapes evenly on the tray.

   Cover the tray with the cloth or screen to keep insects and dust from getting on the grapes.

   Fasten the cloth so it will not blow off.

   Place the tray of grapes in direct sunlight to dry, away from dirt and dust and where air can circulate freely over and under the tray. You may need to put the tray on blocks.

   After 4 days, test the grapes for dryness by squeezing them in your hand. If there is no moisture left on your hand and the grapes spring apart when they hand is opened, the grapes are dry enough. They should then be pliable and leathery.

   If the grapes are not dry, test them again the next day.

   When the grapes are dry remove them from the tray and weigh them. Record the weight. Compare the weight of the grapes before and after drying.

   How much water was lost in the drying process?

   Use reserved grapes for comparisons:

changes in *color*	green to brown
changes in *form*	sphere to flat
changes in *texture*	smooth to wrinkled
change in *taste*	sweet and mild to sweeter and rich

   Eat raisins for a snack. Brush teeth afterward because raisins contain sugar, stick to the teeth, and can promote tooth decay.

   Why are raisins good to eat? They are a good source of iron for healthy blood and provide fiber to prevent constipation.

2. Why do we preserve food?

   to have seasonal foods all year
   to store surplus food for use in times of scarcity
   to be able to transport food long distances

3. How long will the raisins keep without spoiling?

   How long will the grapes keep without spoiling?

   Try an experiment to find out.

Teacher's Note:

Two varieties of grapes, Thompson seedless and Muscat of Alexandria, are used to make raisins. Almost all raisins produced in the United States are made from Thompson grapes. California produces most of the United States' raisins. Other raisin producing countries are Australia, Turkey, Greece, Iran, South Africa, Spain, Cyprus and Argentina. You may want to use a globe and point out these countries and discuss climate in these countries.

Raisins in an air tight container, stored in a cool, dry place will keep in prime condition for more than six months. Grapes will remain fresh in a refrigerator for three to five days.

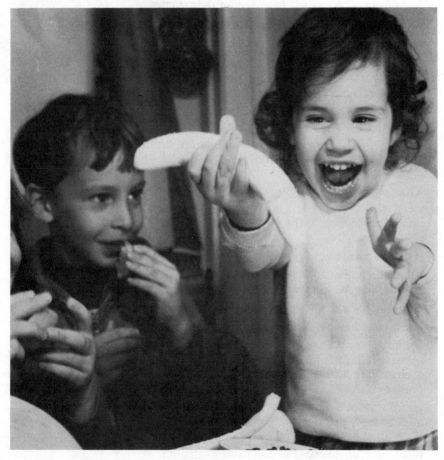

Milk

Milk #1:

Where Do We Get Milk?

Objective:

The children will discuss where milk comes from.

Materials:

Pictures of animals that give milk to people around the world.

Resource section folder, "We All Like Milk", Catalogue, National Dairy Council: Good pictures of female animals and their young

Picture of a mother nursing her baby such as the one found in "Growing Up—How We Become Alive, Are Born and Grow Up" by Karl de Schweinitz (See Resource Section)

Book: *My Friend the Cow* by Lois Lenski

Globe

Make use of experiences that the children or perhaps their friends or relatives have had in other cultures and in other parts of the world.

Procedure:

Ask questions and stimulate discussion:

1. Where do babies get milk? Mothers.
2. Which animals give us milk? Cows, goats.
3. Which animals give milk to people around the world?

   Buffalo—Asia (India, Pakistan), Africa (Egypt)
   Yak—Mountains of Central Asia (Tibet, Outer Mongolia)
   Pien Niu—Mongolia, China
   Sheep—countries around the Mediterranean Sea (Greece)

Goats—Parts of Europe, villages in Greece
Camel—deserts of Africa and Asia
Reindeer—Arctic lands
Horses—parts of China
Donkeys—parts of China

4. How does milk come to us? How does milk get to your house? Use containers to illustrate:

Bags   Cartons
Bottles   Packages
Cans

5. How does the milk go from the cows to the container?

The dairy farmer milks the cows with an electric machine.

The milk is put into a cooler or a refrigerated tank in a special milkroom.

A refrigerated tank truck takes the milk from the dairy farm to a dairy plant in the city.

Have any children ever seen this truck?

The milk is pasteurized by heating it to a certain temperature to kill any harmful bacteria.

The pasteurized milk goes through pipes and is poured into sterile bottles or cartons.

The bottles and cartons are put into containers and placed in refrigerated trucks.

The trucks take the milk to the stores or directly to homes.

(Children will have fun dramatizing this.)

6. What other kinds of milk are available? (See Part 2)

What kinds of milk can you purchase at your school?
    Whole milk, buttermilk, skim milk, chocolate milk.

7. Field trips and resource people:

Dairy farm
Dairy plant
Dairy section in supermarket
Invite the school milkman to the classroom

Teacher's Note:

Although mothers' milk is the best milk for babies, formulas made from cows' milk and soy beans are frequently used.

Milk #2:

Hi Ho The Dairy Oh!
What Is Milk All About?

Objective:

The children will compare some of the different forms of milk.

Materials:

Whole milk—homogenized
Skim milk
Buttermilk
Evaporated milk

Dry skim milk
Small cups
Glass pitchers
Glass bottles

Procedure:

1. Display the different kinds of milk in the containers in which they are purchased.

2. Ask these questions:

   "Are all these forms of milk the same?"

   "Do they look alike?"

   Color: white, bluish or brownish cast, cream color
   Form: liquid, powder
   Consistency: thin, thick, (pour to demonstate), lumpy (buttermilk)

3. Suggest to the children that they smell and taste the various forms of milk.

   Pour about a tablespoon of milk into a cup for each child, using one form of milk at a time.

4. Ask the children to describe aroma, color, taste and consistency of the various forms of milk:

   Smell: Strong, mild
   Taste: Sweet, sour, rich, watery

   Ask: "Which do you like best? Why?"

5. Discuss how the different forms of milk are sold.

   half-pint   half-gallon
   pint   gallon
   quart

6. Practice measurements with dry milk.

7. Dictate, write or draw stories.

8. Use labels and cartons to make collages, mobiles or murals.

Teacher's Note:

Whole Milk—water, milk solids (8.25%) and butterfat (3.25%)

Homogenized Milk—fat uniformly distributed through milk

Pasteurized Milk—see cream line at the top

Skim Milk—milk with butterfat removed

Buttermilk—made by adding culture to skim milk—thick, smooth liquid or the liquid remaining when butter is made

Evaporated Milk—concentrated by removing water from milk, sterilized and canned

Sweetened Condensed Milk—sugar added to concentrated milk (milk with about two-thirds of the water removed)

Filled Milk—combination of skim milk and vegetable fat; or of non-fat milk solids, water and vegetable fat. (The vegatable fat is usually coconut oil, a saturated fat.)

Dry Skim Milk—textured power or granular, made by removing the water from the skimmed milk by spraying the milk on heated rollers

Cream—the part of the whole milk rich in butterfat

A song the class can sing to the tune of "The Farmer in the Dell"

"Hi Ho The Dairy Oh!"
(Use as an action song)

The farmer milks the cow.
The trucks take the milk.
The factory bottles the milk.
To the grocery store it will go.
We all drink the milk.
Milk will make you strong.

Songs paraphrased by Rachel Goodwin, Age 7

Milk #3:

What Can We Do With Milk?

Objective:

The children will investigate some of the products made from milk.

Materials:

Milk	Yogurt
Skim Milk	Cheeses (several varieties)
Cream	Ice Cream
Butter	Toothpicks

Procedure:

1. Let the children see, smell and feel the containers of milk and milk products.

2. Discuss color, temperature, consistency and aroma.

3. Encourage the children to tell about their favorite dairy foods.

4. Discuss how the skim milk, cream, butter, yogurt, cheese and ice cream are made. (See Part I—Page 79, Part 4—Page 83, Part 5—Page 85).

5. Cut the cheeses into cubes and place on toothpicks; let everyone taste the cheese.

6. Taste and compare the variety of dairy products.

7. Ask the children why we drink milk and eat dairy products.
   For healthy bones, teeth and skin.

8. With older children, discuss the key nutrients found in milk and their functions, such as protein for growth, calcium for bones and teeth and vitamins (A , B's and D) for skin, hair and eyes.

Ideas For Other Activities:

1. Other food made from milk—soups, sauces, drinks, puddings and custards. This could be illustrated by food models and pictures. For a special treat make a milkshake.

2. Try a lesson on cheese. Compare the soft and hard ones, the strong and mild ones, the cheeses made from milk, from skim milk, from cream or a mixture of these. Compare natural cheeses and processed cheeses.

Teacher's Note:

Hard cheeses (cheddar, Swiss, etc.) are high in saturated fat, which, in excessive amounts is believed to promote heart disease in some persons. Children should be encouraged to eat cheeses lower in fat, such as cheese made from skimmed or partially skimmed milk.

Milk #4:

Let Us Make Butter And Buttermilk

Objective:

The children will separate milk into butter and buttermilk.

Materials:

Rotary egg beater
Bowl or pint jar with a tightly fitted lid, or individual cups with tightly fitted covers
Small wooden spoon
Measuring cup
Measuring spoon
Knife
Toothpicks for tasting butter
Small paper cups for testing buttermilk
Whipping cream (30% butterfat) (½ pint cream makes ⅓ cup butter)
Salt

Note:

If ripened cream is obtained from a dairy, the buttermilk forms more quickly and will have a tangy taste.

Procedure:

1. Allow cream to come to room temperature.

   Measure cream and put into container, bowl or jar. (Each container should be about half full.)

Beat or shake until lumps of butter form throughout the cream. Everyone will have a turn to beat or shake since 20 to 30 minutes are required to make butter. If the butter is being made in a jar, the class may sit in a circle, pass the jar and count or sing while churning (shaking).

Pour off the buttermilk. Chill buttermilk.

Put butter in a small bowl.

Work remaining buttermilk out of butter with wooden spoon.

Wash butter several times with cold water.

Encourage children to feel the butter.

Taste the butter.

Add ¼ teaspoon salt.

Taste the butter with salt.

Taste butter on homemade bread. Delicious!

Taste the buttermilk.

2. Discuss changes in the cream form: liquid to solid and to a new liquid; cream separated into butter and buttermilk.

   Taste:
   butter without salt tastes sweet
   butter with salt tastes salty
   buttermilk tastes tart

   Color:
   cream-color to yellow in the butter
   white in the buttermilk

   Consistency:
   thick liquid to a soft liquid, to a soft solid plus a liquid

   Texture:
   creamy texture to waxy solid in the butter

3. A song the class can sing:

   "Churn, Churn, Churn the Cream"—Tune: "Row, Row, Row Your Boat"

   Churn, churn, churn the cream.
   Churn, churn, churn the cream.
   Everyone will beam.
   When the butter will be seen.

   Songs paraphrased by Rachel Goodwin, Age 7.

Teacher's Note:

Buttermilk may be made by reconstituting powdered skim milk and adding one half a cup of buttermilk to a quart of the skim milk.

Sour milk may be made by adding one tablespoon of lemon juice or one tablespoon of vinegar to one cup of whole milk.

If a glass jar is used for making butter, instruct the children on the careful handling of the jar for safety.

The butter activity is an important experience. In keeping with reducing the amount of fat intake, use only a small amount of butter. Suggestions for alternative spreads can be found in the recipe section.

Milk #5:

Let's Make Yogurt

Objective:
The children will use a yogurt culture to convert milk into yogurt.

Materials:
First day:

Crock or earthenware bowl
  (1½ quart size)
Measuring spoon
Stirring spoon
Saucepan

Thermometer (optional)
Skimmed milk—1 quart
Culture—4 tablespoons plain yogurt
  (containing live culture)

Second day:

Small cups and spoons for everyone present
Honey and/or fruit in bowls for serving with yogurt

Procedure:
1. Heat milk until warm but not boiling (110° F.).

   Pour into crock or earthenware bowl.

   Cool until a little warmer than lukewarm (test by putting a drop on inside part of wrist; the milk should feel warm but not hot).

   Add yogurt culture (which should be at room temperature) and blend into milk.

   Cover bowl and cover completely with a warm blanket or in a turned-off oven. Let stand for at least seven hours or overnight at room temperature.

   Place in refrigerator.

   The next day put a small amount, about a teaspoon, of yogurt in cups.

   Taste yogurt plain.

   Encourage the children to try more yogurt with fruit or honey.

2. Discuss the change in *form* from a liquid to a solid.
   Taste: Sweet to sour
   Consistency: Thin to thick

3. Older children may discuss which countries use yogurt extensively, why they use it and how it originated.*

Teacher's Note:
For economy and less saturated fat, skim milk made from powdered milk combined with evaporated milk may be used to make yogurt. Reconstitute both according to instruction on can or package. Use about two-thirds skim milk to one-third evaporated. For one quart, use three cups reconstituted evaporated milk plus four additional tablespoons of powdered milk. Proceed as with low-fat milk.

*Yogurt and cheese are ways of preserving milk.

Protein Foods

Teacher's Note:

Meat is a rich source of nutrients, especially protein, iron and the B vitamins. Meat is the most costly food in the diet. The ecological as well as economic costs of producing meat are very high. To produce one pound of meat for human consumption, a steer is fed sixteen pounds of grain and soy.[*] For one pound of meat from poultry, the chicken needs only about three pounds of feed. Cattle, in addition to the low conversion rate, are big polluters. Large amounts of animal waste run off feed-lots and pollute the rivers and streams. *Eating further down the food chain* such as grains, dairy foods, nuts and legumes is ecologically more efficient. The world's food supply would be increased by 35% if we used the land to grow vegetables and grain crops for direct human consumption instead of using it to grow feed for meat producing livestock.

Proteins are classified as "complete" or "incomplete" according to the amount of the eight essential amino acids they contain. Complete proteins are those that contain all the essential amino acids in sufficient quantity and ratio to supply the body's needs. These proteins are of animal origin—meat, milk, (cheese) and eggs. Incomplete proteins are those deficient in one or more of the essential amino acids. They are of plant origin—grains, legumes, and nuts. In a mixed diet, animal and plant proteins complement one another. Grains and legumes also complement each other. Milk, eggs or cheese combined with grains, legumes and/or nuts can provide the correct ratio and kinds of essential amino acids to significantly increase the protein value in the diet. Many Americans consume far more protein than their bodies need, and need not worry much about complementing proteins. However, as escalating meat prices cause a decline in meat consumption, people will seek alternatives, and knowledge of complementary protein relationships will gain in significance.

---

*Cattle are fed grain for a period of time before being marketed; for most of their life they feed on grass.

Summary Of Complementary Protein Relationships

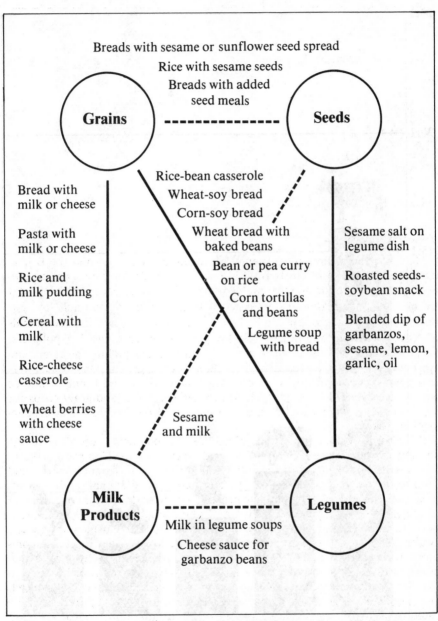

Breads with sesame or sunflower seed spread

Rice with sesame seeds

Breads with added seed meals

Grains - - - - - - - - - - - - - - - - **Seeds**

Rice-bean casserole

Wheat-soy bread

Corn-soy bread

Bread with milk or cheese

Pasta with milk or cheese

Rice and milk pudding

Cereal with milk

Rice-cheese casserole

Wheat berries with cheese sauce

Wheat bread with baked beans

Bean or pea curry on rice

Corn tortillas and beans

Legume soup with bread

Sesame salt on legume dish

Roasted seeds-soybean snack

Blended dip of garbanzos, sesame, lemon, garlic, oil

Sesame and milk

Milk Products - - - - - - - - - - - - - - - **Legumes**

Milk in legume soups

Cheese sauce for garbanzo beans

————————— Complementarity more generally confirmed between several items in each group.

- - - - - - - - - - - - - Complementary relationship demonstrated only between a few items in each group.

Courtesy of Frances Moore Lappé from *Diet For A Small Planet*, Ballantine Books, New York

Livestock Protein Conversion Efficiency

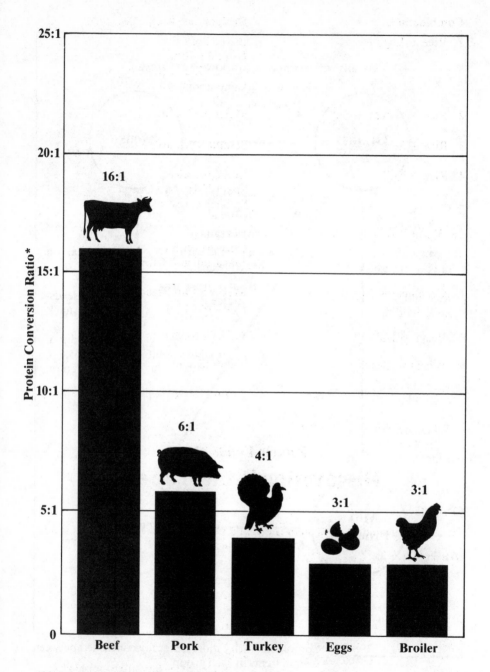

*Number of pounds of grain or soy fed livestock to produce one pound meat for human consumption. (Beef cattle eat grain or soy prior to marketing.)

Courtesy of Frances Moore Lappé from *Diet For A Small Planet*, Ballantine Books, N.Y.

Examples of Complementary Proteins

Combinations	Recipes (See Recipe Section)
1. Rice + Legumes	Baked Split Peas Hopping John Roman Rice and Beans Crusty Soybean Casserole
2. Rice + Wheat + Soy	Mexican Grains
3. Rice + Sesame Seed	Sesame Vegetable Rice
4. Rice + Milk	Con Queso Rice Spanish Rice Au Gratin Spinach Casserole
5. Wheat Products + Milk	Lasagna Cheese Fondue Macaroni and Cheese
6. Cornmeal + Beans	Mexican Pan Bread Pinto Bean Pie
7. Beans + Milk	Bean Chowder
8. Wheat + Beans	Taboulli
9. Peanuts + Milk + Wheat	Peanut Butter Sandwich and Milk

Protein Foods #1:
Discovering Protein Foods

Objective:
The children will discuss protein foods and pair complementary protein foods.

Materials:

Legumes	Dried beans Soybeans Dried peas	Glue Plexiglass cubes or Snap together toys Pictures of milk
Seeds	Sesame seeds Dried corn	Pictures of eggs Pictures of cheese Pictures of beef, poultry and pork

Whole Grain	Wheat
	Rye
	Rice
		Pictures of foods made from
		  complementary proteins
		  (See Teacher's Note)

Procedure:

1. Discuss with children:

    We all like meat. Meat is an excellent source of protein and other nutrients. We probably would not want to give up eating meat.

    Did you ever think about how much land is needed to grow the food (grains and legumes) to feed the steer? The high cost of feeding the steer makes the meat expensive to buy in the supermarket. Would it be better to use more of this land to grow food people could eat? There are many poor people who can't afford to buy the meat.

    What can we do? We could cut down on the number of steers we raise. We could cut down on the amount of meat we eat. We could eat meatless meals and get our protein from foods which could be grown on the land which had been used to grow food for the steers.

2. What foods will take the place of meat? To ensure adequate quality protein for the children, it would be wise to include some animal protein sources in the diet (milk, eggs, etc.)

    Grains + Legumes
    Grains + Milk Products
    Legumes + Seeds

3. Make a protein food matching game:

    Paste either grains, legumes, seeds or pictures of milk or cheese onto the snap together toys, one block for each category, and then snap together complementary protein foods. Complementary protein foods could be glued to matching colors thus making the task self correcting:

    Grains + Legumes should snap together
    Grains + Milk should snap together
    Legumes + Seeds should snap together

Protein Foods #2:

Protein Foods In Other Cultures

Objective:

The children will prepare a fiesta and learn about complementary protein foods in other cultures.

Materials:

Tortillas for everyone	Globe	Cutting board
Tomatoes (fresh)	Knives	Grater
Cheese, cheddar	Plates	Napkins
Taco filling	Bowl	4 Serving spoons
Lettuce	4 Bowls	Saucepan

Procedure:

1. Mexicans have found a way to get complementary proteins in their diet by using foods that are easily produced in their country. Do you know the name of this food? It is a taco.

2. Prepare Tacos. What is in tacos?

   Heat up the taco filling in a saucepan. Use a low temperature. Why? The filling will stick to the bottom and burn. What is in the filling? Read the label or check the recipe. Beans are the main ingredient.

   Divide the children into four groups. Wash and chop tomatoes. Why are tomatoes good to eat? Wash and shred the lettuce. Why do we eat lettuce? Grate the cheese. Why do we eat cheese? Set up buffet style for serving. Heat the corn tortillas. Set food up for a buffet style meal:

   Tortillas
   Taco filling
   Lettuce, shredded
   Tomatoes, chopped
   Cheese, shredded

3. If you have some decorations from Mexico use them—painted gourds, musical instruments, colorful place mats, dance music, lights, etc.

   Have a grand fiesta!

Protein Foods #3: (Nuts)

Nuts For You

Objective:

The children will discover that there are many kinds of nuts.

Materials:

Nuts in shells	Pistachio nuts
Brazil nuts	Peanuts
Macadamia nuts	Hazel nuts
Almonds	Pecans
Cashews	nutcracker

Procedure:

1. Put the nuts in shells in bowls and pass around.

   Have the children describe their size, shape, smoothness, roughness, softness or hardness. Mix them up. Play a naming and sorting game.

2. Crack open several nuts of each kind. Remove them from the shell. Discuss likeness and differences. Taste and smell the nuts. Are they good to eat?

3. Mix up the nuts. Play a matching game by matching the shelled nuts with the unshelled nuts or match the nuts to their shells.

Other Activities With Nuts:

1. Discuss how early man used acorns to make bread and soup. The acorns were dried and ground up between two rocks. The flour was washed to remove a bitter substance. The flour was dried and used for cooking.

2. What animals like nuts? When do they collect them and store them? Plan an outdoor adventure. Look for an oak tree or a squirrel's nest. Watch the squirrels collect and eat the acorns.

3. Do a *fat test* by rubbing a nut on brown paper. A grease spot will indicate the presence of fat.

4. Why are nuts good for your body? Nuts are a good source of protein and a rich source of minerals and vitamins.

5. How could you use nuts in your art work?

Teacher's Note:

Try to use unsalted nuts. If nuts become soft, spread on a cookie sheet and toast in the oven at 325° for 15 minutes. Never use moldy or rancid nuts. Such nuts are extremely hazardous to one's health.

Protein Foods #4: (Nuts)

Peanuts

Objective:

The children will talk about and taste peanuts.

Materials:

Peanuts   Globe or map
(Spanish peanuts:
   raw/roasted/in shell)

Procedure:

1. Do you know where peanuts grow? Look at the globe. They grow in America, China and Africa. In Africa they are called groundnuts. The peanut first grew in South America and was carried by man to the other continents.

2. Do you know where peanuts grow in the United States?

    Georgia, Florida, Alabama area
    Texas, Oklahoma area
    Virginia, Carolina area

3. How do peanuts grow? Plant some and see. The peanut plant produces a flower on its stem above the ground like most other plants. However, it is very unusual. The undeveloped seed travels down through the stem and the pods and seeds develop underground. Peanuts you plant must be raw.

4. What can you do with peanuts?

    Over half the peanuts in the United States are used for peanut butter.
    Salted peanuts
    Peanut oil—used in frying food
    Peanut meal—by-product from the oil used for feeding livestock
    Peanut hulls—shells are used mainly for fuel (peanut shell logs), fertilizer conditioner, poultry litter and livestock feed
    Using all parts of the peanut is good ecology.

5. What do peanuts do for you?

    Peanuts are high in protein for growth and repair of your body.

Peanuts are high in niacin which promotes a healthy appetite and healthy skin.

Both B vitamins, thiamin and niacin, are involved in the release of energy from your food.

Teacher's Note:

Peanuts come in three varieties. There are the runner type, the Virginia type, and the Valencia type.

Peanuts rank among the top ten crops in the United States.

Protein Foods #5: (Nuts)

Let's Make Peanut Butter

Objective:

The children will observe the changes that occur when peanuts are ground into butter.

Materials:

Peanuts (roasted in shells)   Blender
Corn oil   Bowl
Salt   Spoon
Bread or Celery   Spreader
Small plate

Procedure:

1. Discuss favorite ways of eating peanut butter.
2. Have the children remove the peanuts from the shells; remove the brown skins. Observe shell size, shape and texture. Compare the shell with the peanut. What part of the plant is the peanut?
3. Put about 1½ tablespoons of oil in the blender. Gradually add about one cup of peanuts. You may want to sprinkle some batches lightly with salt. Observe changes as the peanuts are crushed and blended into a smooth texture.
4. Serve on bread or stuff the peanut butter into celery ribs.
5. If a blender is not available, you may use a food grinder. The texture of the peanut butter will be coarse and crunchy.

Other Activities:

1. Roast the raw, shelled peanuts on cookie sheets in the oven.
2. Crush peanuts with a rolling pin and add to a salad, soup or bread dough. Also spread on bread.
3. Make peanut butter cookies.
4. What kind of fruit tastes good with peanut butter? Try adding sliced bananas, drained crushed pineapple, raisins, or chopped apple to a peanut butter sandwich.

5. What vegetables do you like with peanut butter? Try lettuce leaf, shredded lettuce, or shredded carrots in a peanut butter sandwich. These are the favorites of some children.
6. Try some peanut butter in your salad dressing.
7. Make spreads from other kinds of nuts or sesame seeds.

Teacher's Note:

If a food processor is available, the addition of oil is not necessary, but the nuts need to be processed beyond the "paste" stage to the "butter" stage.

Protein Foods #6: (Seeds)

Some Seeds We Plant And Some Seeds We Eat

Objective:

The children will discover the seeds that are good to eat.

Materials:

Sunflower seeds   Poppy seeds
Pumpkin seeds   Sesame seeds
Caraway seeds   Anise seeds

Procedure:

1. Are seeds useful to us?

   Seeds are very special. Life comes from seeds.
   Seeds are very good food for us because they are rich in vitamins and minerals.
2. What can you do with seeds?

   Seeds may be planted, sprouted, put on bread, put in salads and eaten for snacks.
3. Which seeds have you eaten?

   In what foods do you like seeds?
   What kind of seeds are good for in-between meal snacks?
4. Have the children taste the pumpkin and sunflower seeds.

   Discuss taste, softness, hardness, size and color.
   Have the children draw pumpkins and sunflowers. Make the sunflowers huge and hang them on the wall.
5. Visit a farm and get a pumpkin. Make a Jack-O-Lantern with a pumpkin.

   Roast the seeds. Sprinkle lightly with salt. They are delicious sprinkled on salad.
6. Make Sesame Seed Squares. See Recipe Section VII.
7. Roast sesame seeds in the oven on a cookie sheet. Crush sesame seeds with a mortar and pestle. Sprinkle lightly with salt. They are delicious when sprinkled on a salad.

8. Sesame seeds, caraway seeds and poppy seeds add variety when sprinkled on breads or cookies.
9. Pumpkin and sunflower seeds are great for snacks.

Protein Foods #7: (Cheese)

Let's Make Cottage Cheese

Objective:

The children will make cottage cheese by separating the curds from the whey using skim milk with rennet or a junket tablet.

Materials:

Collecting bowl or container—4 quart capacity
Double boiler—4 quart capacity
  You can improvise such a boiler with two containers, one large enough to fit inside the other (use stones or clothespins to separate the containers at the bottom). The small container must be large enough to hold 4 quarts.
Draining cloth (cheesecloth).
Junket tablets or liquid rennet.
Pastuerized skim milk, 1 gallon (a gallon makes 1 to 1½ pounds of cottage cheese).
Salt
Bread or whole wheat or graham crackers (enough for each child to have one).
Thermometer

Procedure:

1. Heat water to 80° F. in the bottom part of the double boiler or in the outer container of the improvised boiler. Use a thermometer to determine the water temperature—do not guess at it.
2. Pour the skim milk into the top part of the double boiler or the inner container of the improvised boiler.
3. Dilute 2 or 3 drops of liquid rennet in a tablespoon of cold water and stir it into the milk. If rennet is not available, add 1/8 of a junket tablet to a tablespoon of water and add it to the milk.
4. Allow the milk to remain at 80° F. until it curdles—in about 12 or 18 hours. During this period no special attention is necessary. (The milk may be placed in a warm oven over night.)
5. Place the curd in a drain cloth over a container to drain the whey. Occasionally, pour out the whey that collects in the container so that the draining can continue. In 15 to 20 minutes, the curd will become mushy and will drain more slowly. When it is almost firm and the whey has nearly ceased to flow, the cheese is ready for salting and eating.
6. Salt the cheese to taste. Use as little as possible.
7. Have the children spread the cheese on crackers and taste it.

Teacher's Note:

Cottage cheese is an economical food made of skim milk.

This soft, white cheese is nutritious and can be used as a substitute for meat. Each pound of cottage cheese furnishes as much protein, or body building material as the same amount of beef. However, it does not provide as much energy (calories) as meat, because it it low in fat (made from skim milk).

Curd—The soft, semi-solid part of milk from which cheese is made.

Junket—A preparation of curdled milk and cream that has been sweetened.

Pasteurized Milk—Milk that has been heated to kill bacteria.

Rennet—A substance used to curdle milk.

Skim Milk—Milk with the cream removed.

Whey—The thin, watery part of milk. It is separated from the curd in making cheese. The whey has nutrients and may be fed to birds.

Protein Foods #8: (Cheese)

Let's Make Pot Cheese

Objective:

The children will make cheese by separating the curds from the whey.

Materials:

Unbleached muslin or doubled cheesecloth—½ yard
Strong string, about 1 yard long
1 quart yogurt
Any of the variations below

Procedure:

1. Make a bag with muslin or cheesecloth.

    Hem top, draw string through hem.

    Place about 1 quart yogurt in bag.

    Hang bag by tying to a faucet, or hook over sink.

    Let the whey drip into sink or large bowl overnight.

    Remove cheese from the bag.

    Taste the cheese and the whey.

2. Try some of the following variations:

salt, pepper	garlic
chopped dill	paprika
chopped parsley	caraway seed
chopped nuts	chopped green pepper

3. Discuss the change that occurred in the yogurt:

    Form: a soft thick solid divided into
    a. a liquid—whey
    b. firm solid cheese—curd

Taste: cheese—sweet and mild
     whey—bland

Color: cheese—white
     whey—yellow

Consistency: cheese—crumbly, firm
     whey—thin liquid

Smell: cheese—mild
     whey—mild

Compare: pot cheese made from yogurt with
     pot cheese made from heated skim milk

4. Encourage the children to mix the cheese with favorite herbs, seasonings, vegetables or fruits. Does this change the taste?

5. Use pot cheese for snacks or lunch in sandwiches moistened with salad dressing and favorite variation, or use in salads like cottage cheese.

6. Read Nursery Rhyme: *Little Miss Muffet.* Discuss and dramatize.

Protein Foods #9: (Cheese)
Fondue Party

Objective:
The children will use heat to change cheese from a solid to a thick liquid.

Materials:

Flour—2 tablespoons	Cheddar cheese—⅓ lb.
Corn oil—2 tablespoons	Swiss cheese—⅓ lb.
Milk—1 ⅓ cup	French bread
1 steady fondue pot	Wooden spoon
Fondue forks or toothpicks	

Procedure:

1. Discuss cheese. Where does it come from? Milk or skim milk. What cheeses do you like? Where are they made? Compare likenesses and differences in cheeses.

2. Shred about ⅓ lb. cheddar cheese and ⅓ lb. of Swiss cheese. Cut the French bread into small cubes.

3. Combine 2 tablespoons flour with 2 tablespoons corn oil in a fondue pot. Put pot over flame. Add 1 ⅓ cup of milk. Cook over low heat until creamy. Stir constantly.

4. Add the cheese slowly to the milk mixture, stirring until the cheese is melted.

5. Gather around and put the bread on a fork or toothpick. Dip into fondue. Great for a snack.

6. As the fondue is made, observe the effects of heat on the cheese.

   Consistency: a hard solid to a thick liquid to a soft spread

   Texture: dull to shiny and glossy

7. Put shredded cheese in a cold liquid like milk and observe what happens. Does the cheese change?

Teacher's Note:

Hard cheeses are high in saturated fat, which is known to promote heart disease, so fondues should be infrequent events.

Protein Foods #10: (Beans)

Beans Galore!

Objective:

The children will examine the many varieties of beans—round, flat, little ones, big ones, white, black, green, red, spotted, dotted, fresh and dry beans.

Materials:

Dry beans	Black-eyed peas (beans)
Lima beans	String beans
Pinto beans	Bowls
Turtle beans	Muffin tins
Kidney beans	Paper

Procedure:

1. How many kinds of beans do you know? How do you eat beans? You can boil them, bake them or fry them. You can put them into casseroles or soups.
2. Put the beans into bowls, play with the beans, mix them up, sort them, pour them and use them for measuring.
3. Talk about how they grow. Plant them, sprout them and string them to dry.
4. Where do beans come from? They are grown around the world. Have the children ask their parents or grandparents where they lived when they were growing up and what kind of beans they ate. Perhaps a child's parent or grandparent can come to class to help the children prepare an ethnic bean dish.
5. In summer, try using fresh raw green beans for a snack. Show the children the stem and how the stem attaches the bean to the plant. Remove the stem before eating.
6. How do beans help us grow? Beans are rich in proteins, vitamins and minerals.

Teacher's Note:

Recipes (see Recipe Section) which can be prepared with the children for lunch:

Boston Baked Beans
Chile Con Carne
Three Bean Salad

98

Soybean Snacks

Objective:

The children will see how dried beans absorb water.

Materials:

Soybeans	Bowl
Corn oil	Cookie sheet

Procedure:

1. Put a cup of soybeans into a bowl and wash thoroughly.
   Remove imperfect beans.
   Cover with water.
   Soak in the refrigerator overnight.

2. Next day, compare the dry beans with the beans that have been soaked.
   Observe size, shape, color and hardness.
   What makes the difference?
   The dried beans have the water removed by heat or sun drying.
   The beans that soaked have absorbed water.

3. Drain the beans and spread them out on a cookie sheet.
   Bake at 200° F. for 2½ hours.
   Remove from oven.
   Cool until safe to handle.

4. Drizzle a teaspoon of corn oil over the beans and stir them with a spoon until every bean looks oiled.

5. Return to oven for another half hour.

6. Remove from oven. Sprinkle very lightly with salt.

7. Cool and eat as you would any nut.

8. When thoroughly cool, store in covered jars.

9. How is the soybean used in other cultures?

   Examine samples from an oriental store.

   Several samples are:

   Tofu, soybean curd
   Tamari soy sauce, used in place of salt and other seasonings (high salt content)
   Soybean paste, made with barley and rice (used in a soup eaten at breakfast)

Cereals & Bread

Cereals and Bread #1:

Wheat Comes Out Of The Earth

Objective:

The children will see how wheat grows.

Materials:

Kernels of wheat	Pot of earth
Bowl	Colander or sieve
Water	Towel or cheesecloth

Procedure:

1. Have the children place about ½ cup or more of wheat seeds (kernels) in a bowl.

   Allow enough space for six times the amount used.

   Wash the kernels and soak overnight.

2. Next day, pour the soaked kernels of wheat into the colander in a single layer.

   Put the colander in a bowl and cover with cheesecloth or a towel to exclude the light.

   Keep the kernels moist, dark and dry.

3. Three or four times a day, remove the towel and rinse thoroughly with cool running water.

   This keeps the kernels moist and helps flush away bacteria and fungi which may cause spoiling.

4. Compare the wheat seed before and after sprouting.

5. Taste. Use in a salad or make sprouted wheat bread.

OR:

Plant wheat seeds in a pot. Cover with earth and then water. Each day see if the shoots are above the soil. When the wheat is about one to two inches high, cut and use in a salad.

Cereals and Bread #2: (Cereals)

Cereals—The Staff Of Life

Objective:

The children will investigate different cereals.

Materials:

Choose from this list:

Wheat	Buckwheat
Oats	Grape-Nuts (granulated)
Barley	Shredded wheat
Rice	Puffed rice
Corn	Cheerios (extruded cereal)
Rye	Corn flakes
Millet	Rolled oats

8 small bowls
Pictures of as many of the above as possible growing. See Resource section or write to cereal and bread companies.

Procedure:

1. Put each grain in a separate bowl.
   Encourage the children to feel each grain.
   Mix them up and sort them out.

   Cereal grains are dried seeds or the fruit of cultivated grasses. They are wheat, oats, barley, rice, corn, rye and millet. Buckwheat, although not a true grain, can be ground into flour or used as a cereal. One or another variety may be grown almost anywhere on the earth.

2. Ask the children to name some of the breakfast foods made from cereal grains. Which are your favorite cereals?

   Shredded wheat from wheat
   Rolled oats from oats
   Barley cereal from barley
   Puffed rice from rice
   Corn flakes from corn
   Rye bread from rye
   Millet cereal from millet
   Pancakes from buckwheat

3. What other products are made from cereal grains?

   Baked products—breads, pastries, cakes

Milled products which usually have the germ and bran removed such as white rice, white flour, corn meal, pearled barley, breakfast cereals.

Whole grain products which use the entire grain. They include rolled oats, brown rice, popcorn, shredded and puffed grains, breakfast foods and home ground meals made from wheat, corn, sorghum and millet.

Some beverages are made from grain products such as postum and others from fermented grain such as beer.

4. Have the children match the pictures of the breakfast cereal with the cereal grains.

5. Taste and discuss which of the above cereals are granulated, puffed, shredded, rolled, extruded, or flaked.

6. Why do we eat cereals?

Discuss misleading cereal advertising on television.

Discuss the plusses and minuses of heavily sweetened fortified cereals.

The cereals most advertised are usually highly refined, have excessive sugar added, and are expensive—big profit makers for the manufacturer.

The mineral and vitamin content depends on where they were grown, the conditions of storage and the portion of the kernel used.

Whole grains are a good source of fiber important for preventing constipation and possibly certain diseases of the colon.

Milled or refined cereals have almost no fiber.

Whole grains are rich in B vitamins, trace minerals and vitamin E.

Milling results in a significant nutrient loss.

Enriched cereals have some of the three B vitamins and iron restored or added, but many other nutrients are not restored.

Fortified cereals contain nutrients not normally found in grains.

Some breakfast cereals have added artificial coloring, artificial flavoring, and anti-oxidants called BHT and BHA. Not enough is known about most of these additives. They are suspected of being hazardous to the body.

7. *Supermarket Game*—for older children

Have the children take cereal boxes to school for the following shopping game:
   a. Children shop for:
      cereals without sugar added
      cereals with sugar added
      cereals without color added
      cereals with color added
      cereals which are the most nutritious (whole grain or fortified)
      cereals with added nutrients
   b. Have a discussion about the hazards of too much sugar and unnecessary food coloring.
   c. Encourage the children to dramatize what different kinds of cereals do for them or to them, such as:
      Nutritious cereals give them "Go" power.
      Highly sugared cereals may produce cavities in their teeth.

Grinding Wheat To Make Flour

Objective:

The children will see the change from wheat seeds to flour.

Materials:

Wheat on sheaf
  (available at florist shop)
Kernels of wheat
Flour
Cracked wheat
Bran
Wheat germ

Wheat grinder
Sieve or sifter
Bowl
Microscope (optional) or
  Magnifying glass
Globe or map (optional)

Procedure:

1. Examine with the children wheat on the sheaf.

   If a magnifying glass or a microscope (older children) is available, use it to look at a grain.

   Use a globe or map to discuss where wheat is grown.

   Older children may make a map highlighting the Red River Valley, Iowa, Nebraska, Kansas, and Texas.

   Discuss how the wheat is *thrashed* to separate seeds or grains from the straw or husks.

   Discuss how it is *winnowed* to separate the chaff from the grain.

2. Put the kernels of wheat in the wheat-grinder—an inexpensive grinder resembling a large food grinder—or use a blender (small amounts).

3. Have each child take a turn putting in the wheat and turning the handle of the mill.

4. Sift the ground wheat. Use the coarse part for cereal (cracked wheat) and the flour for making bread.

   Discuss the color and texture of the ground wheat.

   Sift the flour and compare the color and texture of the wheat which does not go through the sifter with the flour that is sifted out.

   What part of the wheat is permanently in the sifted flour?

   What part of the grain is in the coarser wheat?

   The bran and germ may be ground very fine by larger, more powerful mills.

   What is the difference between white and brown (whole-wheat) bread?

5. Show the children the different parts of the wheat.

   The germ has the most food value.
   The bran has the second largest amount.
   In whole grain cereal, all of the wheat is included.
   In refined cereal, the bran and wheat germ are removed.
   In enriched bread and cereal, some of the vitamins and minerals are put back in. (See Cereals and Bread #2)

6. Explore with the children how early man ground his wheat, barley, millet and oats with rocks.

Maybe they would like to try this.

Teacher's Note:

The ancient Egyptians were the first to cultivate wheat. This put an end to their nomadic way of life. The Spanish brought wheat seed to America.

Wheat berry—is the entire grain of wheat.

Germ—embryo or seedling plant within the grain. Most of the nutrients are in the germ and bran layer.

Bran—coat of the grains and associated tissue.

Endosperm—the starchy interior of the grain.

For a free poster on grains of wheat, write:

Kansas Wheat Commission
1021 North Main
Hutchinson, Kansas 67501

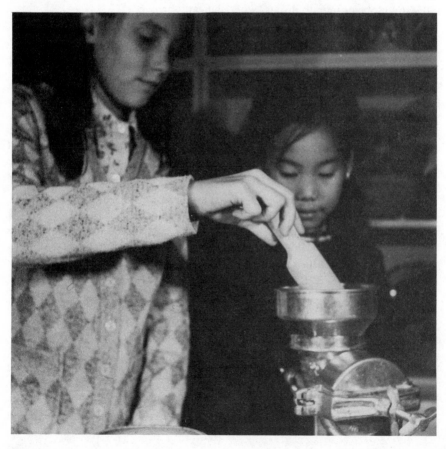

Cereals and Bread # 4:

Let Us Make Cereal

Objective:

The children will see the changes which occur when ground wheat or oats are made into cereal.

Materials:

Cracked wheat (coarse ground wheat) or rolled oats
Powdered milk—¾ cup
Water—3 cups
Nuts, apples or raisins—½ cup
Salt—½ teaspoon
Honey or brown sugar (optional)
Milk
Double boiler
Wooden spoon
Individual cups or bowls
Individual spoons

Procedure:

1. Put 3 cups boiling water in the top of a double boiler and set over the bottom part containing water at medium heat. Be Very Careful.
2. Examine the wheat or oats.
3. Stir 1½ cups of cracked wheat or rolled oats in very slowly to prevent lumping. The cereal should be coated with water. What happens when a small amount of the wheat or oats is added? What happens when a large amount is added?
4. Stir in ¾ cup of powdered skim milk and add ½ teaspoon of salt.

   Observe what happens when the wheat and milk are added to the water.

   Color—milky, cloudy

   Consistency—watery, thin
5. Cook over hot water until thick. What happens if the cereal is cooked over direct heat? Cereal burns and sticks to the bottom of the pot if the temperatur is too high.

   What happens as the cereal is cooking? The cereal is absorbing water, swelling up with water, and becoming a thick mixture.

   Compare the cereal before and after cooking.
6. Add ½ cup raisins or chopped apples or nuts.
7. Serve in bowls. Add a small amount of honey or sugar, if desired.

   Cover with milk. Enjoy it!

Teacher's Note:

Cereal contains some amino acids, milk contains other amino acids, together they form complete protein. A complete protein has all the essential amino acids for humans. Cereal and milk should be eaten together for the maximum benefit. Protein is essential for growth and repair and for the formation of antibodies to fight infection. Protein also supplies food energy.

Take a trip to a grist mill. See "Taking Trips With School Class", Section IV.

Cereals and Bread #5:

Flour Power

Objective:

The children will examine some of the properties of flour.

Materials:

Whole wheat flour—hard and soft
Iodine
Water
Bowl
Baking pan
Aluminum foil

Procedure:

1. "Hard" wheat or "soft" wheat, which is it?

   Have the children squeeze flour in their hands. If it holds its shape it is soft wheat. If it falls apart it is hard wheat.

   Have the children rub the flour between their fingers. How does it feel? Hard wheat feels coarse and granular, soft wheat feels smooth. Flours milled from hard wheat contain firm, elastic gluten, making it especially good for yeast bread.

2. Perform the starch test.

   Put a few drops of iodine on a small sample of flour.

   Observe. A deep blue color results. This is a good way to determine if a substance contains starch.

   Use a potato, cornstarch, sugar, or salt and see what happens.

   CAUTION! Be sure to destroy samples. Iodine is toxic if ingested in this form.

3. Perform the gluten test.

   Gluten enables bread batters and doughs to hold the leavening gas, producing lightness in bread. Wheat flour has the most gluten.

   To examine some of the properties of gluten, form balls of dough from the hard whole wheat flour and the soft whole wheat flour by slowly adding water to ½ cup of the flour until a stiff dough consistency is achieved.

Knead the dough constantly under a stream of cool running water. Kneading develops the gluten. Washing removes the starch. After thorough washing, the water which runs through the dough will be clear and the mass of dough remaining will be crude gluten. Shape the gluten from the hard wheat and the soft wheat into smooth moist balls, put on a pan and bake in a hot oven (450°F.) for one hour. The heat produces steam so the gluten will expand, then become firm. Compare the *size, texture* and *color* of each gluten ball.

To help the children distinguish between the balls before baking, have 2 of the children cut shapes out of foil on which to place the gluten balls; perhaps one ball could be placed on a round, flat bread shape and the other on a loaf shape.

Teacher's Note:

Depending on the age of the class, resources, etc., whole wheat flour gluten galls (hard and soft) could be compared to rye, soy and/or buckwheat flour gluten balls.

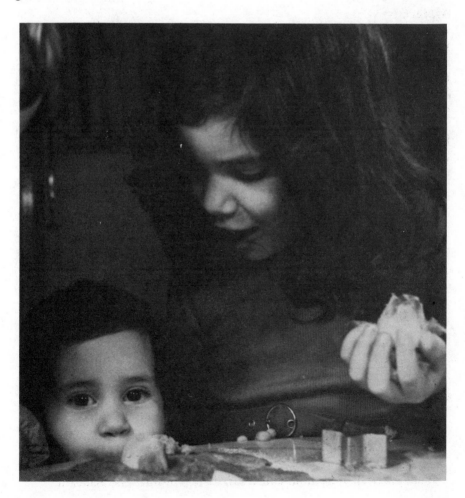

Let Us Make Bread— Great Expectations

Part I

Objective:

The children will see and discuss how important bread is to man.

Materials:

Breads or pictures of breads from many lands.
Bread molds
Utensils used in the past or in other cultures

Procedure:

1. Discuss: What is bread?

   Bread may be as simple as a combination of flour, water and salt, baked in an oven or over an open fire.

   Today, bread is made this way in parts of India and Africa.

   In the southwestern part of the United States, certain Indian tribes still make their bread this way.

2. Whenever man has baked bread, he has considered it a magical and sacred process, a medium for expressing himself.

   The first bread was made in China or Egypt.

   The Chinese fermented and steamed their bread.

   The Egyptians were the first to discover that if they let the dough sour or ferment before baking, it became raised bread which is the forerunner of our "sour dough".

   Columbus carried "sour dough" starter in the hold of his ship when he came to America.

   The first public bakeries were in Greece.

   The French Revolution was ignited by a bread riot.

   "Buckwheat Cakes" were made famous in London by James Whistler.

   In frontier America, women baked bread in skillets in front of their kitchen fires.

   Bread made from meal and water and baked in a pan was called "corn pone". When this same dough was covered with ashes and baked in an open fire, it was "ash cake". When the dough was baked on a hoe over a fire, it was called "hoe cake".

   "Johnny Cake" was an American Indian bread, sometimes called "Journey Cake", because it was often carried by travelers.

Pancakes or griddle cakes were called "flannel cakes" in American lumber camps. This name was developed in honor of the flannel shirts worn by the lumbermen.

3. Bread is the staff of life to people all over the world. How many breads of other lands do you know?

India—Chapatti	France—Pain Ordinaire
Pakistan—Nan	Ireland—Irish Soda Bread
Russia—Koulitchey	Italy—Grissini
Scotland—Scones	Israel—Challah, Pita
England—Biscuits	Japan—Pan
Mexico—Tortillas	China—Men Pau
Sweden—Limpa	Middle East—Pita

4. Bread is important as a ceremonial food. Do you know any ceremonies involving bread?

During the dark ages, the art of bread baking was kept alive in the monastaries.

For some Christians, special bread is used for communion. Catholics call this bread "hosts".

The Romans and Greeks held bread sacred and sacrificed bread as images of their gods.

In ancient times, Egyptian bread was a symbol of truth. Persons took a sacred oath with their right hand touching the top of the loaf.

Jews use special flat bread for Passover called matzos.

Orthodox Russians have special bread for Easter called Koulitchey.

In Latin America on All Soul's Day, the dead are remembered by bread offerings which are taken to the cemeteries. Similar gifts are made by the living and given to each other.

In Germany, St. Nicholas Day is celebrated with a sweet dough made into the shape of his helper, Peter, carrying a bundle of twigs.

In Scotland, a relative of the bride is expected to break a bun over the head of the new wife before she sets foot over the threshold of the new home.

In Sweden, the bride and groom eat a whole wedding bread to symbolize a faithful and happy marriage.

In ancient Syria, the people sprouted wheat on plates or in jars in their homes. At the start of the new year, the young shoots were taken to a river or lake and cast into the water. This custom is "casting bread on the water" to return as answers to prayers.

Would you like to create your own ceremony based on what bread means to you?

5. Today, bread companies may be brought to court for misleading nutritional claims about their products. Continental Baking Company, a subsidiary of International Telephone and Telegraph (I.T.T.) agreed to a consent order by the Federal Trade Commission for advertising Profile Bread as a diet bread, containing fewer calories per slice than other breads. The company was required to run corrective advertisements disclosing that Profile

109

Bread had fewer calories per slice because it was sliced thinner than the other breads.

Discuss TV ads for popular breads. What do the ads imply? How much nutritional information do they convey?

Wheat and bread supplies are a major international issue. Those who control the production and distribution of wheat and other basic food crops control, to a large extent, who lives and dies on this planet.

These are good topics of discussion for older children.

Teacher's Note:

Visit international food shops and see how many different kinds of bread you can find. Discuss what they contain and how they are made and used. Compare likenesses and differences. Visit a bakery.

Cereals and Bread #7:

Let Us Make Bread— Great Expectations!
PART II

Objective:

The children will see what ingredients are needed to make bread and how it is made.

Materials:

Flour—main ingredient. How many different kinds of flour do you know?

Liquid—milk, buttermilk, fruit juice, vegetable water, water

Salt—adds to the taste in the bread

Yeast—tiny plants which multiply rapidly when moist and warm. A small amount of brown sugar or honey will provide food for more rapid growth of the yeast.

Oil—adds flavor, makes the bread tender; peanut butter may be used for oil.

Egg—adds nutritive value, flavor, and helps the bread to rise. Aids in leavening.

Sugar—small amounts of honey, molasses or sugar may be added for flavor and to make the bread tender.

Other ingredients—spices, herbs, seeds, cheese, fruits and nuts may be added.

Procedure:

1. What kinds of bread do you know?
   Yeast breads—loaves, rolls or flat breads, Pita or Nan
   sweet breads

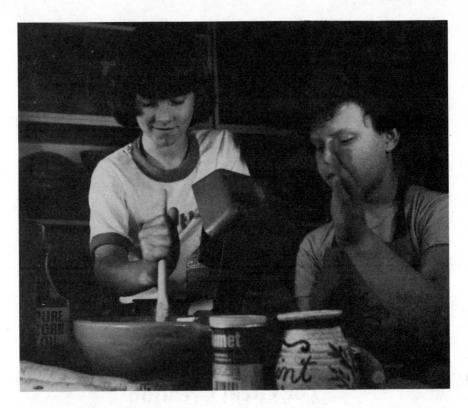

sour-dough breads
rye, whole wheat, white, oatmeal
kasha, potato bread
Unleavened breads—matzos, cornmeal (palenta)
Quick breads—loaves, muffins, scones, biscuits, popovers, corn bread, spoon bread, pancakes, waffles

2. Why is stirring, beating, and kneading so important in bread making?

Wheat flour has special properties which make it preferable for most breads.

When liquid is added to the flour and the mixture is beaten, stirred or kneaded, a substance called gluten is formed.

Gluten enables the bread batters (thin mixtures) or the dough (stiff mixtures) to hold the leavening gas, producing the "lightness" in breads.

Kneading develops the gluten.

Flour from other grains may be mixed with the wheat flours.

3. What is the yeast's contribution to the bread?

The tiny yeast plants, a biological leavener, grow with moisture, warmth and a small amount of sugar.

Too much sugar slows down the yeast growth.

As the yeast plants grow, they produce a gas called *carbon dioxide*.

The carbon dioxide gas bubbles throughout the flour mixture and makes the dough light and porous.

In quick breads a chemical leavening agent is used.

Children may enjoy acting this out through creative dramatics and dancing.

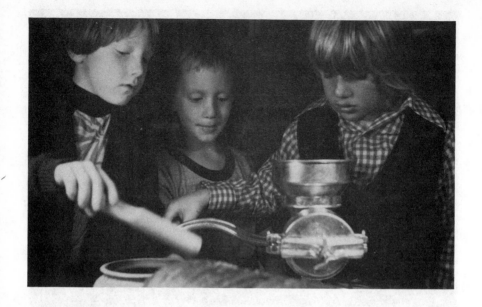

Cereals and Bread #8:

Let Us Make Bread— The Great Creation
PART III
(Discussion suggested in Part II may be incorporated into Part III)

Objective:
The children will make flour into bread.

Materials:

Whole Wheat Flour—3 cups
Corn Oil—2 tbsps.
Milk—1 cup
yeast—1 package
Brown Sugar or Molasses—¼ cup
Salt—2 teaspoons
Boiling Water—½ cup
Lukewarm Water—½ cup

Large mixing bowl
Measuring spoons and cups
Wooden spoon
Saucepan
Cup
Medium mixing bowl
Baking sheet
Tube pan, round with hole in center

Procedure:

1. Have the children wash their hands very carefully.
2. Use the numbers and quantities for math concepts.
   Put into mixing bowl:
   1 package of yeast
   ½ cup lukewarm water
   Let stand for 5 minutes.

3. Put in a separate bowl:
   1 cup milk
   ½ cup boiling water
   ¼ cup molasses or sugar
   2 teaspoons salt
   2 tbsps. corn oil
   Mix well, cool to lukewarm (wrist temperature).

4. Add yeast to mixture.

5. Stir in:
   3 cups flour
   Beat well with heavy spoon. When dough becomes stiff, mix with hands. If sticky, add a little more whole wheat flour.

6. Knead until the dough is smooth and elastic (about 8 to 10 minutes).

7. Put dough in an (oiled) large mixing bowl. Oil the dough and cover with a clean towel.

8. Place in a warm place and let rise to double bulk (about 1 hour).

9. Shape into loaves, rolls or imaginative shapes.

10. Try making a face, an animal, masks or special designs with dough.

11. You may want the children to make foil flags with their names and stick them into their masterpieces with toothpicks before they go into the oven. Shapes change during raising and baking. Do you like the fragrance of bread baking?

12. For a grand celebration, have the children oil a tube pan. Have each child shape the dough in round balls the size of walnuts. Fill the tube pan two-thirds full with the balls. Proceed as for bread. Save this loaf for the grand celebration.

13. Decorate the bread with seeds, nuts or dried fruits.

14. Place in oiled baking pans. Put in a warm place. Cover with a clean towel.

15. Let rise to double in bulk (about 50 minutes).

16. Bake loaves about 50 minutes, rolls about 20-30 minutes, at 375 °F.

17. Encourage children to participate in every step.

18. How does the batter, dough, bread, look, feel, smell and taste?

19. Is it fun to make a loaf of bread?

20. What are your favorite shapes?

21. Why is wheat called the staff of life? Whole grains are important to our diet because they have:

    (a) Many B vitamins:
        —important for being alert
        —for steady nerves
        —and a good appetite

    (b) Minerals like iron to make our blood and our whole body work better.

    (c) Fiber to keep us regular and prevent constipation.

    (d) Protein which helps build and repair our bodies.

    (e) Starch for energy.

22. What happens as the bread bakes? The yeast is killed by the heat. The liquid in the bread is converted to steam and expands the gluten, raising the bread.

23. Remove bread from pan and cool on a rack. Encourage each child to admire, take pride in his or her creation. Have the children talk about how the bread looks, feels, and smells and compare the bread with the dough.

24. Taste and see how good homemade bread is. How does it sound when the child bites into the crusty, chewy crust? How does this differ from store-bought bread?

Refrigerator Dough:

1. Dough may be prepared one day and shaped and baked up to 4 days later.
2. Double yeast if dough is to be refrigerated.
3. Dough may be refrigerated after kneading or after rising. If allowed to rise, it would need to be punched down.
4. Oil well and cover with a clean cloth or bowl.
5. When the dough is removed from the refrigerator, it may be kneaded and shaped immediately or allowed to come to room temperature (2½ to 3 hours).

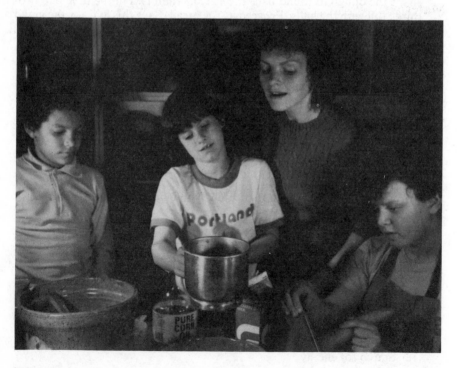

English Muffins:

1. Use bread dough that is ready to be shaped.
2. Remove dough the size of an egg and pat into rounds about ⅓-inch thick on a well-floured surface. Cover and let rise to double in bulk.
3. Lift muffins on to a hot, lightly greased griddle with a spatula, very gently or they will fall. Be very careful or you may get burned.
4. Fry slowly for 15 minutes, turn and fry for 15 minutes on the other side.
5. Tear apart with a fork and toast, serve with cheese or your favorite spread.

Cereals and Bread #9:

The Magnificent Feast

Objective:

The children will taste and celebrate the breaking of bread.

Materials:

Their own round loaf of bread
A candle for the center
A beautiful bread board
Knife
Butter, margarine or cheese
Small plates and spreaders for everyone
A pleasant, attractive setting befitting their masterpiece
Very special guests

Procedure:

1. The round bread celebration may take place the following day.
   Heat up the bread if desired.
2. Plan a party.
   Tell stories about bread, sing songs, dramatize bread making yesterday and today.
3. Create a beautiful atmosphere for the work of art.
   Maybe a tablecloth, colorful napkins, flowers or wheat in a ceramic pot on the table.
   Use things from nature for decorating.
   Have a display or poster of the process from wheat to flour to bread.
   The Egyptians painted murals about bread making. Maybe you can also.

4. Consider a parade around the class or the school with the bread.
   Older children may carry a lighted candle in the center of the bread. Be very careful!
   Use home-made musical instruments and perhaps write a song for the parade.
5. Come back to the class and pass the bread around for each person to break off a piece and celebrate together.
6. Encourage discussion about the bread experience. The creation of bread deserves respect and appreciation by all.

Teacher's Note:

The atmosphere in which children eat may be as important as the food. Today's life style has led to eating on the run, without the time to savor a good meal or good food.

Cereals and Bread # 10:

The Festival of Breads

Objective:

The children will talk to different people about bread making and breaking.

Materials:

A teacher who can make things happen.
Children who have discovered the meaning of bread.
Parents who want to create a beautiful celebration.

Procedure:

1. Have the children interview their parents, grandparents and neighbors, especially those from different ethnic backgrounds or other countries.
   Have the children find out what kinds of bread they ate as children, what kinds of grains were used, how it was made and how it was eaten.
   Was the bread used for any family or community ceremony?
2. Have the children report and share their stories.
3. Compare bread then and now.
4. Collect some new bread recipes.
5. Have a bread making festival at the school.
   Have interested families make bread from their ethnic backgrounds.
   Children need roots and identity in our homogenized society.
   Food is a marvelous way of relating family history and giving children a sense of belonging.
   A. Plan a fair and at this fair involve family members in bread making demonstrations out of their own backgrounds.
   B. At the fair, have plays on the history of bread or on family customs involving bread.

C. At the fair, have a contest for the most nutritious and delicious, the most creative and imaginative bread.

D. Plan a ceremony at this fair which involves the community in the breaking and sharing of bread.

E. Celebrate with folk songs and dances. Wear dress appropriate to the country of the origin of the bread.

6. The Museum of Contemporary Crafts in New York had an exhibition on breads—*The Baker's Art*—in 1966.

It is time for your school or community to have one, too.

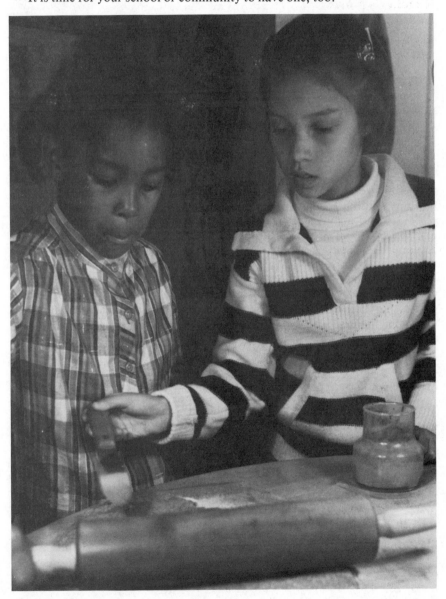

More Fun
with Food Learning
Experiences

Let's Make Ice Cream

Until a few years ago, ice cream was a very special treat made for family celebrations, church socials and county fairs. Today it is fashionable to turn sweets into the mainstay of the diet. A good example of this is the "High Protein Breakfast Cake", a highly fortified cake with a cream filling and often a frosting. This has been used in some school breakfast programs.

At one time, cake was considered a treat for birthdays and other special occasions. Ice cream and cake should be considered "extras", and not a main part of the diet. Ice cream is not equivalent in nutrients when compared to milk. One hundred calories of milk has significantly more nutrients than one hundred calories of ice cream. This is due to the much higher fat and sugar content in ice cream.

Objective:

The children will convert milk from a liquid to a solid, ice cream, by freezing and observe the changes.

Materials:
Ice Cream#1

Freezer for making ice cream	3 eggs
Bowl	2 cups brown sugar
Rotary egg beater	1 teaspoon salt
Measuring cup	2 15-ounce cans evaporated milk
Crushed ice—6 quarts	2 quarts milk
Coarse rock salt, 1 1/2 cups	2 teaspoons vanilla

118

Procedure: Ice Cream #1

1. Break eggs.
   How do they look, feel, taste, smell?

2. Beat eggs.
   What happens to the color, shape, amount and consistency as you beat?
   Air is incorporated into the egg mixture, increasing its volume.
   Beat in sugar and salt.
   What is occurring? Is the mixture the same consistency?

3. Stir in the vanilla and milk.
   How does this addition affect the consistency and color?

4. Pour into a gallon-size freezer cannister.

5. Pack freezer with crushed ice and add coarse salt to ice, alternating ice and salt in about three layers.
   Observe the crystals in coarse salt. Compare coarse salt and fine salt.

6. Make ice cream by turning the handle slowly at first, then more rapidly.
   Turning the handle incorporates air into the mixture, resulting in a lighter, smoother ice cream.
   Smoother ice cream has small crystals; coarser ice cream has larger crystals.

7. As ice settles or melts, add more ice and salt.

8. The ice cream should be ready in 15 to 25 minutes.

9. Because the ice cream may be soft, you may want to freeze it before serving.

10. Taste to see how good the ice cream really is!

Variation, if desired: Add chopped nuts or chopped fruit.

Ice Cream#2

2 pans that fit inside each other, or	3 eggs
2 metal bowls that nest inside each other	2 cups brown sugar
Metal spoon	1 teaspoon salt
Crushed ice—4 quarts	2 15-ounce cans evaporated milk
Rock salt	2 teaspoons vanilla

Procedure: Ice Cream #2

1. Ice cream may also be made by using a large pan of ice, sprinkled with coarse salt.

2. Beat eggs.

3. Beat in sugar and salt.

4. Stir in milk and vanilla.

5. Put a small amount at a time of this mixture into the second pan.

6. Place the second pan on top of the ice.

7. Stir as the ice cream mixture freezes.

8. The change from a liquid to a solid can be observed.
9. This will make soft ice cream.
   The soft ice cream may be served as is, or frozen hard by putting into a freezer.
   A. Discuss when, why, and what happens when liquids freeze.
   B. Observe the changes which occur when a liquid changes into a solid.

Form:	liquid—can be poured
	solid—holds a shape
Consistency:	thick or thin
Texture:	smooth or coarse
Temperature:	which is colder?
Taste:	same or different?

   C. If both ice creams are prepared, compare:

Weight:	light or heavy (depending upon amount of air incorporated)
Texture:	smooth or coarse
Taste:	strong or mild flavor—delectable!
Consistency:	soft or hard

Teacher's Note:

A fun celebration is an Ice Cream Social. For a special treat, make vanilla ice cream. Have an assortment of fresh fruit, nut, honey or granola toppings. Encourage the children to make their own sundaes.

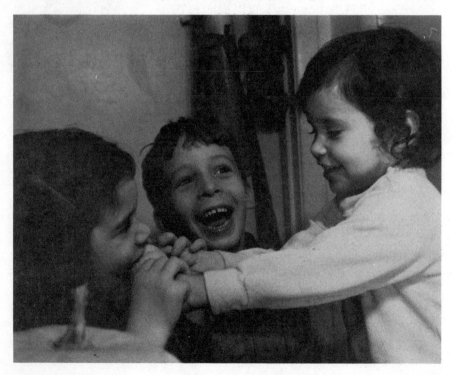

Let's Celebrate With A Birthday Party

Objective:

The children will have a birthday party with the bread and other foods.

Materials:

1 unsliced loaf of bread
4 different kinds of sandwich fillings
   (cheese, eggs, chicken, cole slaw)
Cream cheese
Green pepper
Cherry tomatoes
Milk/Juice
Home-made musical instruments
Construction paper
Glue

Balloons
Songs
Poetry
Felt pens
Tray
Knife
Spreaders
Plates, cups and forks for everyone

Procedure:

1. Celebrations are a marvelous way to express love for others.
   To celebrate a child's birthday is to tell the child, "We are happy you exist."
   Make a child king or queen for the day.
   The day before the party, have the children make crowns or hats out of construction paper.
   Have each child contribute something personal to the birthday child such as a poem, a song, a picture, a flower, or a good wish.

2. Prepare a sandwich loaf by removing the crust from the bread.
   Slice the bread lengthwise, making five layers.
   Have the children spread a layer of filling on four layers.
   Stack them and place the fifth on top.
   Soften the cream cheese, add a little milk, if necessary.
   Cover the sandwich loaf with cream cheese.
   Decorate it to look like the child's favorite toy.
   Use pepper rings, quartered cherry tomatoes, parsley, carrot sticks and curls for trucks, trains, flower baskets, names, etc.
   Chill the sandwich loaf.

3. Blow up balloons, write the name of each child on the balloon with a felt pen, or write a good wish to the birthday child, or have each child draw his favorite design.

4. Have a parade wearing the hats.
   Play the musical instruments, sing, dance, dramatize a happy event.

5. Gather around the table, slice and serve the sandwich loaf, pour the milk or juice and serve. Paper cups could be decorated with cut-out designs.

6. The birthday child could be the host or hostess.
7. Have the children present their gifts.
   If the class is large, try a birthday party for all the children born in a specific month.
   A theme for the month could be picked such as springtime—new life, fall—harvest, etc.

Food Choices and Lifestyles

Objective:

The children will discuss and express themselves as to how they feel about the food they eat, how they eat it, and why they eat it.

Materials:

Newsprint	Cardboard
Paint	Magazines with food pictures
Brushes	Labels from favorite foods
Paste	Scissors

Procedure:

Discuss with the children:

1. How was food grown many years ago?
   It was grown on small farms and in private gardens.
2. How is most of our food grown today?
   Huge companies own and control the production of our food from the seed to the table. Trace a company's activities growing, processing, storing, packaging, transporting and selling food.
   Is the company local or national?
   What kind of advertising does the company do?
   What brands are advertised?
   Surveys have shown that children's favorite brands remain favorites into adulthood. Thus, advertising promotes brand loyalty.
3. Who is producing the food for your community? Small farmers? Large corporations or both?
4. How has this affected our eating habits?
   We eat fewer natural, homemade, and ethnic foods.
   Food is less interesting.
   Convenience foods are bland and rob the cook of opportunities to develop meals creatively and imaginatively.
   Convenience foods encourage members of families to eat at different times.
5. Would you enjoy a family garden or potted herbs growing in the kitchen window?
   From your garden or your window box, you could help to create artistical-

ly a beautiful table and add to the family's enjoyment of a wonderful dinner as the family discusses the events of the day.

6. How many times a week do you think the family or friends should eat together? Is this possible within our hectic, modern lifestyles?

7. Recognizing that family members are very busy and that convenience foods, drive-in restaurants, vending machines, etc. allow us time to get many things accomplished, do you feel such food habits should be a way of life?

8. What are some of the unusual foods, regional foods, homemade foods, homegrown foods, ethnic foods, etc. you most enjoy?
   From the discussion, do you think there is too much sameness in the eating habits of all of us?

9. Make collages or paint pictures of:
   a. foods which have special meaning to you.
   b. foods from specific geographic areas where you have lived.
   c. foods you have grown.
   d. foods with which you associate good memories or positive emotions.

10. Do you buy food for yourself and/or your family?
    Do you prepare it or help prepare it?

Teacher's Note:

Reinforce self reliance and independence. Keep track of whether or not the children have changed their eating habits and their food likes and dislikes as the food unit continues. Build on good food selections; raise alternatives for poor ones.

Suggest that children keep a record of:
   the kinds of foods they eat in a hurry at home.
   what comes out of a vending machine.
   what is available at a fast food restaurant.

Invite parents and the class to make a pot luck lunch for all to enjoy, to plan, prepare and serve at school featuring favorite or special foods. Have the youngsters arrange and set the table and make place cards as well as assist in the preparation.

Take a field trip to and eat at a place where all of the food comes out of vending machines. Discuss what it would be like to eat like this every day.

Have older children write stories about the origin of foods, food choices, lifestyles or the meaning of food to them and to others.

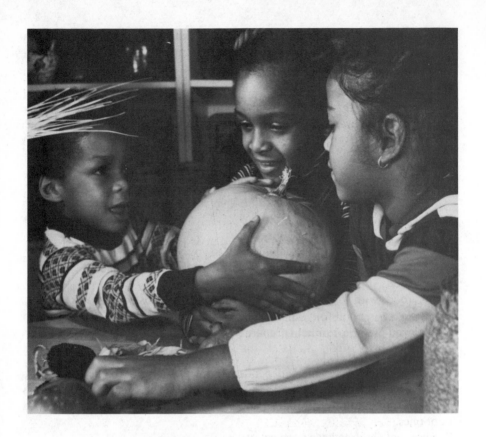

To Market, To Market,
In Search of Good Food

Objective:

The children will go to market to investigate the variety, quality, and quantity of nutritious foods available. See "Taking Trips With School Class"—Section IV.

Materials:

Supermarket

Procedure:

1. The supermarket can be a living museum for the creative teacher.
   For each food category studied, you may find that a trip to the supermarket, a natural food store, an ethnic food store or a country market would greatly enhance the children's knowledge of food. Today, many children shop for food.
   Supermarket field trips should focus on how to select good food buys.
   Older children may find unit pricing, open dating, and nutrition labeling of interest.
   Ask for the supermarket's consumer specialist to give you a tour.

2. Prepare for the field trip. Discuss with the children:

How much space is allotted to wholesome foods, to junk foods, to non-food products?

Are some foods or food products manufactured primarily for good nutrition while others are manufactured primarily for profit? Do some food companies market wholesome food and other companies market junk foods? Check brand names and see.

What kind of food displays are at the ends of the aisles, near the door, check-out counters, and at other conspicuous places at the eye level of children? What is their purpose?

Which foods do parents buy on the request or demand of their children? Why do children want these foods?

Which foods offer prizes or other gimmicks?

Which foods are packaged to tempt children?

Set up a supermarket in the classroom. Have the children bring empty containers from home. Perhaps the food service in the school could provide some assistance.

3. Suggestions for supermarket tours.

Overview of the supermarket:

Have the children identify the areas where the nutritious foods are displayed (dairy, produce, legumes, lean meat, fish, bread, cereals).

How much space is allotted to nutritious foods; count the rows or shelves. How much to junk foods? Is there a section for non-food items? Outline a floor plan with each section identified.

Overview of a natural, ethnic food store or a country market:

Follow the procedures as above. Compare differences in food availability, variety, quality, and price.

Discuss with the children: Dairy Products

What kinds of milk are available? Whole milk, skim milk, buttermilk, 2% butter-fat milk, chocolate milk, evaporated milk, dried milk.

What kinds of cheese are available? Natural, processed. See what coloring and preservatives are added. Look for the origin. Observe cheese foods and cheese spreads. Read label for content. What fillers and additives are used? Compare cost with natural cheese.

What type of artificial dairy products are displayed? Creamers, whips, etc.

What forms of dairy products are available? Fresh, canned, dehydrated.

List the best buys.

Discuss with the children: Fruits and Vegetables

What are the differences in the variety, quality and origin of available fruits and vegetables?

Are seasonal ones less expensive in season?

Is color added for cosmetic reasons? Florida oranges and red potatoes may be dyed.

Was the produce picked by unorganized workers or poorly paid migrant workers? Which companies have unions and which ones do not?

The produce is available in what forms? Frozen, fresh, canned, dehydrated.

How has the produce been processed? Has it been waxed?

How many artificial fruit drinks are displayed? Who manufactures them? What do they contain? Look on the labels for the words methyl cellulose, artificial, imitation, synthetic.

Discuss with the children: Protein Foods

What are the variety, quality and origin of legumes, nuts, meats, fish, and eggs?

What forms of legumes are displayed? Canned, dried, etc.

Which fish are shell fish? Which are fresh water and which are salt water fish? In what forms are they available? Whole fillets, steaks (raw or cooked), fresh, frozen, canned, dehydrated, smoked.

What different cuts of meat are available? Are they lean or high in fat, fresh, frozen, smoked, cured? Compare the prices of processed meats such as bologna, hot dogs, etc. to other protein foods. Processed meats are probably the poorest in nutritional value and dollar value of the protein foods.

Make a list of the best buys.

Discuss with the children: Bread and Cereal

What are the variety, quality, sources and origin of whole grain, enriched and unenriched cereals and breads?

How much of the grain ingredient is whole grain?

How much is white? Is color added? Ingredients are listed in order of decreasing amounts. The first ingredient listed is present in the largest amount.

Compare weight and size of loaf. The soft breads may be puffed up with air.

Check the manufacturer of each kind of bread.

Which cereals have sugar, coloring and preservatives added?

Which cereals are junk foods? Which ones are nutritious and are not debased by excessive sugar, saturated fat and potentially harmful food additives.

Which cereals have nutrients added?

Make a list or collage of labels of the best buys.

Teacher's Note:

The following books may be of use in understanding our present food situation and what can be done about it:

The Supermarket Handbook: Access to Whole Foods, Nikki & David Goldbeck; Harper & Row, New York, 1974

Nutrition Scoreboard, Michael Jacobson; Avon Books, New York, 1975

Better Living Through Better Eating, Mary T. Goodwin, Montgomery County Health Department, Rockville, Md., 1974, rev. 1979.

The Hidden Persuaders, Vance Packard; McKay Publishers, New York, 1957.

The Limits To Satisfaction, an essay on the problem of needs and commodities: William Leis, University of Toronto Press, Toronto and Buffalo, 1978.

What Is Your School Food Service Program Doing For You?

Objective:

The children will evaluate the school food service program.

Materials and Resources:

School lunch menus
School breakfast menus
Cafeteria Manager

The legislative intent of the school food service program is to safeguard the health and well being of the nation's children by serving nutritionally adequate lunches and coordinating the schools' health education activities with the formation of good eating habits in the lunchroom. Participating children will gain a full understanding of the relationship between proper eating and good health.

In 1978 the regulations were revised. Proposed changes were made for amounts of food for specific ages. Contact the U.S. Department of Agriculture, Director, School Food Programs Division (Washington, D.C. 20250) for the current regulations.

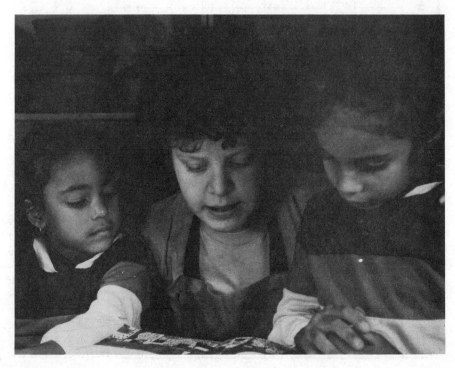

Proposed School Lunch Meal Requirement*

Daily Lunch Pattern	Pre-school 1-2 Yrs	Children 3-4 Yrs	Elementary 5-8 Yrs	School Children 9-11 Yrs
1. Protein Foods—One of the following foods or a combination to yield equivalent quantities of protein:				
Meat, poultry, fish, cheese	1 oz.	1 1/2 oz.	1 1/2 oz.	2 oz.
Eggs	1	1	1	1
Cooked dried beans and peas	1/4 cup	1/4 cup	1/3 cup	1/2 cup
Peanut Butter	2 tbsp.	2 tbsp.	3 tbsp.	4 tbsp.
2. Vegetables and/or fruit	1/2 cup	1/2 cup	1/2 cup	3/4 cup
3. Bread	5 slices/wk.	8 slices/wk.	8 slices/wk.	8 slices/wk.
4. Milk, whole, skim, buttermilk	3/4 cup	3/4 cup	1 cup	1 cup

*The following changes in the school lunch program were effective as of August, 1979:
(1) expand the list of bread alternates to include enriched or wholegrain rice, macaroni, noodles, other enriched or whole-grain pasta products, and other cereal grains such as bulgur and corn grits; (2) require schools to serve lowfat milk, skim milk, or buttermilk; (3) require School Food Authorities to devise a program of student involvement; (4) require School Food Authorities to devise a program of parent involvement; and (5) recommend that schools which do not offer a choice of foods serve no one form of meat or meat alternate more than three times a week.—*Director, School Programs Division, USDA-FNS, Washington, D.C., (202) 447-8130.*

School Breakfast Pattern For All Children

1 cup milk—whole, skim, buttermilk
1/2 cup fruit or full strength fruit or vegetable juice
Whole grain or enriched bread or an equivalent serving of cereal, cornbread, biscuits, rolls, muffins or 3/4 cup of cereal, pancakes or waffles

As often as possible:

Protein-rich foods such as an egg, a one-ounce serving of meat, poultry, fish, cheese, or 2 tablespoons of peanut butter.

Procedure:

1. Draw up menus using the Type A Pattern for hot lunches, cold lunches (salads, sandwiches) and a hamburger platter or breakfast menus for schools with or without cooking facilities.

   Consider color, texture, flavor and form.

   Are there foods for cleaning the teeth and stimulating the gums?

   Do the menus have foods containing fiber, such as whole grains, raw fruit and vegetables?

   How many calories and important nutrients are in the lunch?

2. Do the students creatively participate in planning, preparing and serving the school meals?

   Student committees on school food service can be valuable if they are given realistic guidelines and reasonable suggestions are implemented. Students could learn food service skills useful for summer jobs and part-time employment.

3. Is a variety of nutritious foods, seasonal foods, and regional foods frequently served?

   A wide variety of nutritious food is more likely to provide the essential nutrients; various fruits and vegetables contain different kinds and amounts of nutrients. Use of regional foods may give students a sense of belonging and help support small local farmers who would supply fresh foods and more variety than the international corporate conglomerates. Natural foods are best.

4. Take a field trip to the cafeteria at lunch time.

   Observe:

   • Is the lunchroom atmosphere pleasant?

   • Describe the aroma coming from the lunchroom. Smell is an important part of food enjoyment.

   • Is the Type A lunch well prepared and attractively served?

   • How many children buy a Type A lunch?

   • Are the children who don't buy a Type A lunch eating a balanced lunch?

• Do they bring lunch from home or buy a la carte items at school?

• Do the Type A lunches meet the federal guidelines? Is there a choice of foods in the Type A lunch? Choices provide opportunity for decision making.

Today's children have to take more responsibility for their own health than in the past. They need to be given the opportunity to make decisions which will benefit their health. Availability is one of the most important factors in food selection.

• Are the meals carefully selected to provide a wide variety of wholesome foods?

About 60 known nutrients are important for human nutrition. A diet con-containing a wide variety of natural foods is best. Raw fruits and vege-tables, and whole grain bread and cereal contain fiber. Foods high in fiber promote healthy teeth and gums as well as a healthy colon.

• Is the food carefully prepared?

The foods selected and prepared should provide a variety of nutrients and a variety of colors, textures, flavors and forms. Hot foods should be served hot and cold foods served cold. If food is overcooked and mushy, not only does loss of taste and appeal result but nutrient loss occurs also.

• Is the food attractively merchandised?

The eye eats first. If the food looks good, the chances are the students will taste it.

• Are junk foods served at the same time and place as the Type A lunch? If so, why?

• Do the students have more junk food to select from than wholesome foods?

• Are *a la carte* items competing with the school meals? Bombarding child-ren with a variety of junk foods may undermine their health. Educational institutions should be setting an example and not encouraging children to eat foods that are debased by excessive amounts of sugar, saturated fat and potentially harmful food additives. Fabricated, formulated, fake foods are making huge inroads into institutional feeding.

• Is the school kitchen closed and preplated meals substituted for meals prepared on site?

Closing school kitchens is closing alternatives. Preplated lunches are in-ferior in nutrition, taste, texture, and color to meals prepared on site. In addition, some foods used are diluted with extenders and others are laced with food additives. Little is known about the additive, accumulative and synergistic effects of many food additives.

• Are throw-away plastics, paper and aluminum containers used in serving the meals?

A recent study published in the *Journal of the American Dietary Associa-tion* shows it is cheaper to use and purchase dishwasher and reuseable dinnerwear. Disposable items also may undermine children's feelings of security and for the world around them. Our resources are not unlimited. The ecological ramification of throwaways is far reaching. Consider the value system that is being encouraged in children.

- How much food is thrown out?

About one-half of the U.S. population eats an inadequate diet. Some of these are the over 25 million Americans who are poor and probably hungry. In general, it is estimated that about 400 million people around the world go to bed hungry. At your school, run an experiment by measuring wasted food in gallon containers. How many people would the wasted food feed? How much does the wasted food cost? Try to determine the reasons for wasted food. Conduct interviews to find out why foods are thrown away. Some possibilities are poor menu choices, poor preparation and unattractively presented food. A rushed atmosphere may invite waste as well as the use of disposable plates, a negative attitude by the staff toward the food or the children, a lack of awareness of the importance of food, etc.

- Is more than 10 percent of the food served wasted?

Try an archaeology study and measure the waste. What is the cost of the food wasted? How many people could be fed with this food. What is the educational message? Why is the food being wasted? Consider the high cost of food, the world food shortages, and world famine.

- Do the students have adequate time to eat and savor their food (20 to 30 minutes)?

When students are rushed and hurried, there is a tendency to waste food and a negative attitude toward eating may result.

- Is the environment in the cafeteria pleasant and relaxing, and the attitude of adults conducive to enjoyment?

The environment in which students eat may be as important as the food. A noisy or regimented atmosphere may result in rejection of food. A pleasant atmosphere is far more conducive to development of good eating habits.

- Is the food offered under psychologically acceptable conditions with proper regard to the students' self-respect?

If positive emotions are aroused, the program is contributing to the emotional well-being of children. If negative emotions are aroused and the meal is unenjoyable, the lunch program may be detrimental to the child's self-respect. Eating and being fed are intimately connected with one's deepest feelings. Food offered without due regard for childrens' self-respect may result in their disliking school, thereby poisoning their relationship to school and learning.

- Do the teachers eat the same food as the students? If the teachers have different food from the students, one may suspect that it is not good enough for them, perhaps a suggestion of classism.

5. Does your school have a vegetable garden?

Vegetable gardens could provide food for its cafeteria and for classroom demonstration, as well as an opportunity for students to learn gardening skills and provide worthwhile contact with nature.

6. Does your school have celebrations?

Children love celebrations. Why not have community celebrations of special people or famous people in your community, events or holiday with a local festive flavor. Both the school and the community could be involved in the planning, preparation and celebration. This is a great way to foster a sense of belonging to a community. (Perhaps even reduce vandalism.)

7. Does the school administration feel the school food service makes an important contribution to the growth, development, learning and behavior of the children?

8. Present the findings to the administration. If your school has a fine food service program, encourage the children to commend the administrators. If the program is poor, involve parents in expressing concern over the importance of a good program. Have them assist in trying to improve the program. Work out a plan for change involving all concerned.

Teacher's Note:

Nutritive Value of Foods, U.S. Department of Agriculture, Government & Public Section, 14th and Independence Avenues, S.W., Washington, D.C.

Eating Better at School, Center For Science In The Public Interest, 1755 S Street, N.W., Washington, D.C. 20009. $2.00.

WHAT IS THE MESSAGE?

Objective:

The children will analyze the advertising messages directed at them on TV, in magazines, on trucks, in the supermarket, etc.

Materials:

TV ads   Children's magazines
Food labels   Delivery trucks
Trip to supermarket

Procedure:

1. Discuss with the children the purpose of highly intensive marketing via television directed at children.

The average child watches 25 to 30 hours of television per week. This is more time than the child spends in the classroom.

In one year the moderate TV-watching child potentially sees between 8,500 to 13,000 food and beverage commercials.

Between 400-600 million dollars a year is spent on television advertising of food and drink directed at children. The largest component of advertising specifically directed toward children is for sugared foods such as pre-sweetened cereals, candy, and cookies. Excessive consumption of sugar contributes to the development of tooth decay and possibly to other problems such as obesity and its health consequences. It also lays the roots for a child's long-term preference for sugar in the diet at the expense of nutritious foods. Television advertising for sugared foods discourages the child from learning sound nutritional habits and skews his/her concept of what good food really is.

Children are highly vulnerable to intensive advertising. They have considerable spending power through badgering adults into buying advertised products. Children are particularly susceptible to developing brand loyalties and they are the consumers of the future.

The consequences of supporting a highly consumptive culture leads to a prodigal, spendthrift, extravagant and wasteful society.

2. Have the children watch TV on Saturday morning and after school.

Ask them to observe the TV food commercials carefully.

Ask the children to count how many advertisements they see or hear on food from delivery trucks, billboards, radio, TV, etc. in one day.

Have the children act out the commercials. If products are available, use them.

What is the overriding message?

Remember all advertising appeals are not verbalized.

The purpose of advertising is to sell, promote consumption.

Consider how many (if any) of the products advertised are necessary or useful.

What claims are being made?

Is a premium or membership an enticement to purchase?

Is a leading sports personality, news personality, entertainer or any familiar cartoon character or favorite storybook character used in the commercial?

Are children used as spokespersons or employed to deliver the sales message?

Are empty calorie products, or products debased by excessive amounts of sugar, saturated fat and potentially harmful food additives advertised?

Is a synthetic food advertised in such a way as to imply that it is comparable to or made from a natural food, such as an orange "flavored" drink advertised as orange juice?

Are claims made directly or by implication that any edible product or nutrient by itself produces, hastens or enhances vigor, stamina, strength, energy, growth, intellectual performance?

Can these claims be supported by facts?

Are these foods protective to health or potentially harmful to health?

Bring in labels of the products and read the ingredients.

If ingredients are not listed, write the manufacturer to find out what they are.

What type of food habits are being promoted?

What food companies promote products consistent with good food habits?

What values are the commercials emphasizing?

Are they emphasizing positive values that should be reinforced or values that may be personally or societally destructive?

3. Have the children work out and dramatize their own commercials for wholesome foods.

Teacher's Note:

In his book *The Limits to Satisfaction,* William Leiss states that "the increased number of commodities has created a unique social culture in which marketing is the main social bond. Values no longer shape and condition needs, wants, drives, or preferences." The major emphasis placed on increasing the Gross National Product has resulted in highly intensive marketing practices to promote the use of commodities. Advertising is used to create "needs", "wants" or "desires" for these products. This leads to an increased confusion in determining and satisfying needs. Liess states that "the underlying dynamic (is) the systematic orientation of all needs toward commodities. This situation promotes a lifestyle that is dependent upon an endlessly rising level of consumption of material goods." Individuals are thus led to misunderstand the nature of their needs and the ways in which they may be satisfied. As the variety and number of commodities increase and highly intensive advertising promotes consumption, needs escalate but become harder to satisfy. This lack of satisfaction leads to fragmentation and alienation. Society as a whole suffers from the excessive exploitation of resources. Putting our children in the forefront of this consumptive destructive effort through advertising is not only disgraceful but tragic. A tape or video tape of a commercial would be useful. Older children may write to the FTC (Federal Trade Commission), their Senators and Representative, and local newspaper and TV stations to express their views on TV commercials aimed at children.

Children's Advertising
Federal Trade Commission
7th and Pennsylvania Avenue, N.W.
Washington, D.C. 20580

Let the food manufacturers know what the students think about their advertising. For information on advertising budgets of the food industry see "Advertising Age" September 6, 1979.

Film:

"Supergoop" by Churchill Films available from:

Food and Nutrition Information Center
U.S.D.A., National Library of Agriculture
Beltsville, Maryland

IV. SUGGESTED ACTIVITIES FOR EXPANDING THE SCHOOL FOOD AND NUTRITION CURRICULUM

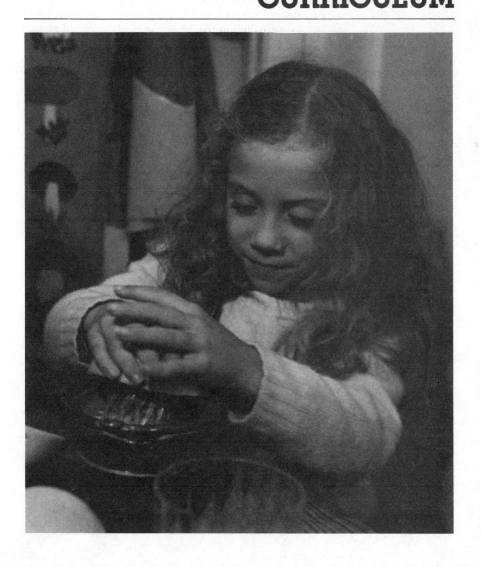

Developing
Language Skills

Teacher's Note:

Most of the activities children take part in should build language skills.

1. Word Identification:

Play Food Lotto (Bingo): Proceed from simple food identification and classification according to groups (fruits and vegetables) for younger children to food families (citrus) and complementary foods for older children.

Decorate the room with food pictures and encourage the children to identify the foods. Pictures of more exotic foods and more detailed food charts might challenge older children.

Bring in and talk about many different kinds of foods.

Play fishing: Make fishing rods out of sticks, string and dime store magnets. Attach paper clips to construction paper food shapes or magazine pictures. Children identify those foods that they catch.

2. Discussions:

During a group sharing time, encourage general conversation relating to food and the daily routine. Remind the children that each person will have a turn to speak.

Talk about what each one does when one gets up in the morning, before one goes to school, during school, after school, in the evening. Encourage them to remember which foods they ate at different times of the day and whether or not it was time for breakfast, snack, dinner, etc.

Use pictures and books to expand discussions. Make a collection from magazines or use sets which can be purchased. Try to include not only pictures of foods but also those depicting people marketing, the preparation of food, people eating at a table together. If possible, find pictures with children in them. Don't forget farm pictures and pictures of children planting seeds. Pictures, slides and films of foods and peoples from around the world would stimulate good discussion for older children.

Help the children "read" the pictures. You may ask them some guiding questions, but then let them tell you what they see. Do not give them words unless they ask, but use good descriptive words yourself as you speak to them. Your words should refer to size, shape, location, color, etc.

Ask them what *their* favorite foods are. Suggest that they bring pictures of foods into school to show to the class.

3. Experience Charts and Memory Games:

After cooking or baking with the children, review with them what was done and what was used. Perhaps this would be best done the next day.

Use the utensil chart again. Let the children identify the utensils.

Play *What Happened Next?* Give the children clues if needed or just guide them as they go over the sequence of cooking steps.

Have the children dictate or write a *Cooking Experience Chart* which you or they print on a large piece of paper. Illustrate and post where the children can read it.

4. Using Descriptive Words As Clues:

Play *What Am I?* "I'm long, orange and crunchy when I'm eaten raw. What Am I?" (a carrot)

5. Word Sounds:

Play rhyming games. What fruit rhymes with bear? You could use a picture of a bear or just say the word. How many words rhyme with pea?

Call attention to initial sounds. How many words or how many foods can you think of that begin with the same sound as the "c" in corn?

You can do this with final sounds also. Pictures help children remember while they are thinking.

Find food names inside other words. Which food do you see in the word "acorn"?

Developing the Senses

1. Visual Skills

Play *Food Lotto (Bingo)*

Make a food shape chart with matching cards.

Have the children find the shape that is different, such as three apples and a banana.

Play What Doesn't Belong?

a) Out of four pictures, one is not food

b) Out of four pictures, one is not fruit

c) Out of four pictures, one is not a protein food (for older children)

Play What Is Missing?

Show the children four foods or pictures of the foods.

Have the children close their eyes while you take one away.

Ask them to tell you which one is missing.

Let the children take turns removing one while the others in the class keep their eyes closed.

You might use a flannel board if you are using pictures.

Play Sequence Patterning.

Arrange in sequence two, three, four or more foods or food pictures.

Ask a child to reproduce the foods or pictures in the same sequence using your sequence as a model.

With some experience, the child might try to reproduce a sequence he/she has seen from memory (no model).

Ask the child to set up a sequence pattern for you to reproduce.

Play Picture Memory Game.

Show the children a picture related to food or their daily routine.

Hold it up for a few seconds and then take it down.

Ask the children to tell you something about the picture they just saw.

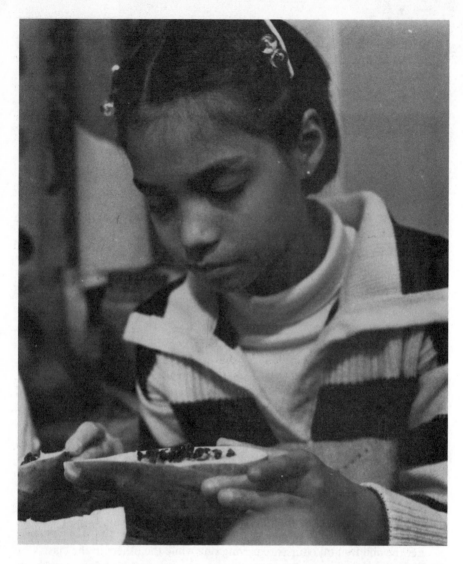

2. Have children observe a variety of foods using all their senses.
(Sharpening the senses is important for people of all ages.)

Seeing

Identify foods by shape, form, color, texture.

Is it curved, is it straight?

Does it grow separately or in bunches?

Does it look the same on the inside as on the outside?

Does it have sections?

If it is a fruit, how many seeds does it have?

Is it juicy or dry?

Use words like pulp, rind, pod, glossy, dull, dark, liquid, fluffy, solid, shiny, light, fresh, stale.

Classify foods according to their color.

Hearing

Listen to the sounds made as different foods are eaten.

Listen as food is being cooked. What does boiling water sound like, or popping corn?

Play a guessing game with eyes closed. How many food sounds can you identify?

Ask for descriptive words such as crunch, crackle, etc. Children can be very imaginative.

Touching—texture, temperature, weight

Is it hard or soft, hot or cold, heavy or light, rough or smooth?

Allow the children to feel the differences but suggest only one descriptive word at a time so that you do not confuse them.

Hide food in a drawstring bag and ask the children to identify the food by feel.

Blindfold an older child or ask a younger child to close his or her eyes and let the child sort beans or nuts by feel.

Scoop out a pumpkin and separate the seeds for roasting.

Use words like sticky, crisp, grainy, solid, smooth, soft, hard, rough, coarse, waxy, prickly, slippery.

Smelling

Have children smell many different foods.

Herbs and spices are excellent for sharpening the sense of smell.

Have children try to identify foods by smell with their eyes closed.

Use words like pungent, sweet, sour, bitter.

Alert children to cooking and baking aromas.

Tasting

Give children opportunities to taste salty foods, sweet foods, sour foods, bitter foods and bland foods.

Encourage children to tell you how the foods taste. They should hear your descriptive words, but you should accept their descriptive words also.

Play a guessing game by having children close their eyes and try to guess what you feed them.

Use words like crisp, delicious, burnt, pungent, strong, sharp, mild, spicy, nutty, peppery.

3. Comparison of foods which look similar in pictures.

Children sometimes confuse the apple and the tomato in pictures.

Bring a real apple and a real tomato to school and study the differences.

Bring a lemon, a grapefruit and an orange into school and talk about how they are alike and different.

You could even add a lime to the discussion.

Lettuce and green cabbage is another possibility for comparison.

The class could also prepare two varieties of the same food such as red cabbage and green cabbage, or red apples and green or yellow apples.

Have different varieties of lettuce available for the children to taste and compare.

Offer the children a small amount of sugar and salt to compare. First by sight and then by taste.

Learning Through
Role Playing

1. **Use books, nursery rhymes, finger plays, songs, dances and puppets to stimulate role playing.**

   Read and encourage the informal dramatization of such stories as:

   > "The Little Red Hen"
   > "Stone Soup"
   > "The Gingerbread Man"

   Sing songs or introduce finger plays which allow the children to act out their daily routine or plant a garden or be a garden.

   Children become seeds, sun, wind, trees, rain, etc. with the slightest suggestion. "Here We Go Around the Mulberry Bush" is a good song for this purpose. There are many others.

   Singing and dancing are important not only because they provide an important means of expression for children, but because song and dance also help children understand new concepts. If the child becomes a growing seed or a rooted tree or a carrot who is proud of his nutritive value, the child relates to this knowledge and it becomes part of him/her. There are many good songs and dances relating to food and health. Others can be adapted to the subject. Research or create with the children songs and dances which dramatize planting, harvesting, preparing foods, eating, etc. The children can either be the food or the plant or the person working with the food or the plant.

2. **Role Playing is a good follow-up after a trip.**

   Following a trip to the market, have the children help you set up a classroom market using cans and cartons from home, a cash register and a few paper bags. Some simple guidance from you as to the role of the clerk and the customer is all the children need. Their imaginations will keep the game going.

3. Role Playing before or after baking or cooking may be helpful.

Play the game of the mysterious yeast.

The group makes a circle.

The children take the parts of the ingredients which are needed to make bread.

When all necessary ingredients are in the center of the circle (the mixing bowl), they are crouched down and huddled together.

Now the child who plays the yeast enters the center and something special happens!

All the other ingredients begin to rise up and move away from each other.

The yeast is added to make the bread rise.*

4. Casually set the scene for free play role-playing.

Don't forget how important the impromptu dinner party or picnic is during free play time or how good the sand box ice cream or cake tastes. Perhaps you could suggest some more nutritious foods for pretend play.

Try to have safe, stimulating kitchen equipment in the housekeeping area.

Make sure role-playing is kept simple, flexible and informal.

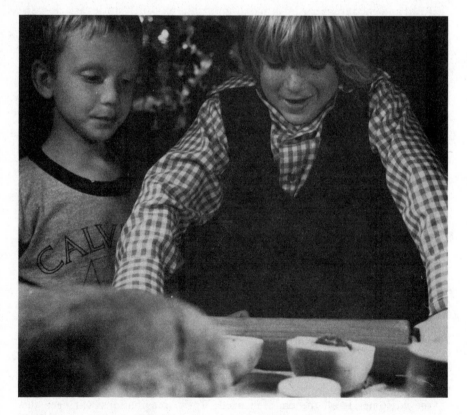

*See Bread and Cereals #7, page 111, for more information on yeast and how it works.

Developing
Mathematical Skills

1. **Give children the opportunity to play with measuring equipment.**

    Provide water or rice or beans or cornmeal in one or more large bowls.

    Add measuring cups, measuring spoons, pitchers of different sizes, funnels, strainers, egg beaters.

    Keep the groups small, allowing each child ample space.

    When playing with or talking with the children, use words such as full, empty, half, whole, how much, how many spoons or cups, level, more, less, through the funnel, strain, beat, mix, pour, etc.

2. **Play money and numeral matching.**

    If a classroom supermarket or food store has been set up, mark the food cans and cartons with numerals you wish the children to be able to recognize.

    Make play money by cutting rectangles out of heavy paper and marking the money with the corresponding numerals.

    The money should be made to fit the cash register or a box and can be used by the children to "buy" the food.

    Older children can add to get the needed amount and "change" can be made.

3. **Use beans and seeds as counters.**

    Play simple counting games, demonstrate 1-1 correspondence, add, sub-Cut or have the children cut approximately 3" x 3" squares of colored tissue paper.

4. **Use real foods to solve portioning problems.**

    Have children decide how they will share a certain number of apples, raisins, popcorn.

Have children decide how they will share a pie.

Suggest that the children take as many carrot sticks as they have pockets or buttons or birthdays.

5. Setting the table.

Allow children to set the table for a specific number of people.

This activity reinforces 1-1 correspondence.

This activity reinforces lateral perception.

6. Measure the children for height.

Repeat every few months.

Put a measuring tape up in the classroom.

7. Weigh the children.

Help them read the scale.

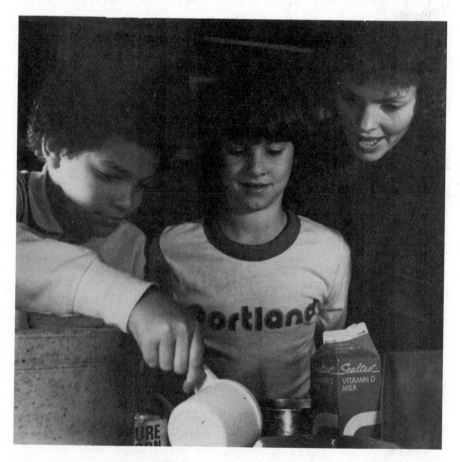

Learning Through
Arts and Crafts

Teacher's Note:

Allow the children to do as much as they can do on each project.

Be as helpful as necessary without doing for them what they can do for themselves.

Don't worry about perfection. Experience in "doing", not perfection, is the goal.

Make sure that the children's tools are safe and in good condition.

Have enough staplers, hole punchers, scissors, etc., so that children are not expected to wait for long periods of time. Enthusiasm doesn't last forever.

Give the children plenty of time and guidance as they learn to use the tools and materials.

Be open minded about the children's suggestions concerning color, choice and construction. Sometimes children see things differently than adults. Don't get "hung up" on realism.

There is some difference of opinion about the use of real foods for arts and crafts projects. Certainly among low income groups, this is an important consideration. Waste should not be encouraged in any classroom. The teacher should use her best judgment in this regard.

1. Use vegetables and fruits to make beautiful prints.

Oranges, grapefruits, apples, lemons, carrots, onions, celery stalks, green peppers, and potatoes make beautiful prints.

Cut fruits or vegetables in half across the diameter or lengthwise.

Dry with paper toweling.

Pencils, plastic spoons, forks or blunt knives may be used by the children to carve a design in the potato.

Paint pads are made by folding pieces of paper toweling, about four folds thick, placing the folded paper into separate dishes or sectioned plates and saturating the toweling with brightly colored paint.

Almost any paper can be used for the printing, even tissue paper.

Fabric or paper may be used to print *table place mats*.

Printed tissue paper makes lovely wrapping paper.

2. Make food shapes from clay or play dough.

Join the children as they experiment with the play dough or clay. *Roll* the clay, *coil* it, *pinch* it, *slab* it. The children will eventually notice and perhaps try their hand at it.

Various foods can be fashioned with play dough or clay, (and painted if preferred) when the children become experienced in the use of the material. Give the children plenty of time and opportunity to experiment.

When ready, the children might make:

fruit baskets

food mobiles—
Show the children how to hang hardened food shapes from wooden or clay dowels or metal hangers using strong nylon thread or yarn. Don't forget to suggest that the children make holes or loops for the thread before the clay hardens. They may need needles in order to pass thread or yarn through the holes.

paper maché food—
Cover the clay shapes with strips of newspaper which have been dipped in liquid starch, or a flour and water paste, and allow to dry thoroughly before painting. Shorter, wider newspaper strips are easier for younger children to handle. Let the children tear their own strips.

3. Some foods make good materials for collaging and stringing.

Macaroni comes in a large variety of shapes and sizes. It can be painted or left unpainted and then glued to paper or cardboard to string on yarn.

Fruit seeds, dried beans, peas and nuts are also excellent for pasting or gluing.

4. Don't forget painting and drawing.

Food can inspire colorful easel painting, finger painting and watercolor marker drawings, especially when decorating a room for a holiday.

Give the children a long strip of paper and markers for a mural.

Let the children decorate a white paper *tablecloth* with markers.

Cut easel paper into food shapes and ask the children to guess what the food may be.

5. Use food to make rhythm instruments.

Put rice or beans in an empty baking powder can, replace lid, paint and decorate.

Buy various shaped gourds in the autumn, allow them to dry out and then listen to the dry seeds inside.

Put rice or beans in a toilet paper roll and then cover completely with aluminum foil.

6. Use magazine and newspaper pictures of food and growing things.

Use the pictures and words for:

food scrapbooks
food family mobiles
collages
food charts
posters illustrating a favorite poem or fingerplay about food or growing things, an animal or plant.

7. Make egg shell glitter.

If desired, the children might color egg shells with vegetable food coloring or paint when dry.

Have the children break the shells with their fingers, or for finer glitter, have them crush the shells with a rolling pin.

Designs are fun to make when the glue is squeezed from the bottle with squiggles and swirls or drawn on with a cotton swab, then the glitter applied, allowed to dry, and the excess glitter spilled off. Young children enjoy watching some glitter fall off while some glitter stays on.

8. Make a turkey for Thanksgiving.

Trace or have the child trace his own hand.

The thumb is the turkey's head and real feathers or feather-shaped papers which have been fringed can be pasted to the body. Fringing paper is a good early cutting activity.

It is best to show the children a good picture of a turkey or a turkey in a film, if they can't see a real turkey. They should be familiar with the turkey's wattle and feathers.

9. Make flowers for a pretty table.

Egg carton flowers:

Cut egg carton sections out separately.

Let the children paint and decorate the egg carton sections.

Make a hole or have the children make a hole in the base of the flower.

The children add the pipe cleaner stem, doubling the pipe cleaner in the hole to keep the flower from falling.

Leaves may be added.

Put "flowers" in a decorated paper cup flower pot.

Tissue paper flowers:

Go for a walk and find some twigs.

Cut or have the children cut approximately 3" x 3" squares of colored paper.

Children can crumple the tissue paper and glue it to the twigs and add paper leaves.

The twigs may then be sunk into clay which has been placed in a can, cup or margarine container. The bottom half of a milk or cream carton also makes a good flower pot.

Weeds and wild flowers.

Pick attractive weeds and wild flowers for your table centerpiece.

10. Make a fruit tree.

Go for a walk and find some nicely shaped fallen branches.

Sink the branches in clay in a shoe box.

Decorate the box and cover it with paper "green grass."

Hang paper, clay, play dough or paper-made fruit from the tree.

Let the children string doubled yarn, nylon thread or string through the fruit with plastic or steel yarn needles.

Have the children add crumpled green tissue paper for leaves.

11. Make a seasonal tree.

Prepare the tree as in #10.

Hang on the tree paper shapes, pictures or clay shapes, representing the foods of the season and other symbols of the season.

12. Decorate an orange juice can for Mother's Day.

An orange juice can covered with construction paper and then decorated with beans, nuts and macaroni or painted designs or yarn, makes a good pencil holder for Mother or Dad.

13. Make Pomander balls.

Cover an apple with whole cloves (stick cloves into apples).

Mix equal amounts of cinnamon and ground orris root (available at drug store).

Roll apple in the mixture, covering well.

Wrap in plastic wrap and allow to dry for several weeks.

Tie with a pretty ribbon and hang as an ornament or hang in a closet for its aroma.

14. Trace the children.

Make a full size tracing of each child on large brown or white paper. Older children can trace each other.

Have children fill in, with crayons or markers, their faces or any other parts of the body they might want to detail. This can be a culminating activity after time has been spent on the concept of self—parts of the body, health and good food, daily routine, feelings, family, etc.

Learning
About Science

1. Making observations:

Observe the veins of a leaf, the stem and the hairs on the roots of a plant under a magnifying glass.

Talk to the children about how the plant gets its water and food through the root hairs and how the water travels to the leaves.

Observe the inside of a lima bean which has been soaked overnight.

Notice that the seed absorbed the moisture and notice how it has changed.

Notice the tiny plant and stored food inside the seed.

2. Seeing likenesses and differences.

Give the children the opportunity to classify nuts, seeds, beans, etc.

Give children the opportunity to categorize foods into groups.

Suggest that the children sort silverware.

3. Finding out what plants need:

Do green plants need water?

Materials:
2 similar potted plants

Procedure:
Place both flower pots in the sunlight.
Water one plant daily. Do not water the other.
After several days, notice that one plant is thriving while the other is wilted and dying.
Water, which is necessary for life, was kept from one plant.
The plant was unable to manufacture its food and began to die.
Try to revive it by watering it.

Do green plants need sunlight?

Materials:
2 similar potted plants   1 large box to serve as a cover

Procedure:

Cover one plant with the large box.

Make several holes in the box to let air in.

Water both plants daily.

After several days, compare the healthy green uncovered plant with the one that was covered.

The covered plant will probably be yellowed and frail.

Sunlight was kept from the plant.

It did not have the opportunity to manufacture its own food (photosynthesis).

The plant suffered from "malnutrition".

Try to revive the plant by placing it in the sun.

Do green plants need air?

Materials:

2 similar potted plants

1 large jar

2 small dishes of water

Procedure:

Place each flowerpot in a small dish of water.

Cover one plant with a jar.

Press the jar into the soil so that no air can reach the plant.

Place both plants in the sunlight.

Observe what happens after several days.

The plant getting the air will show great vitality and life.

We have seen so far that plants need sunlight and air and water.

4. Find out how plants grow:

Do plants bend toward the sun?

Materials:

A green plant

A large corrugated cardboard box

Procedure:

Make an opening in the side of the box about the height the leaves will reach when placed inside.

Place the plant in the box directly in the path of the sun.

After several days, the leaves and stems are bent toward the light of the sun.

Turn the plant so that the leaves point away from the opening.

After several more days, they will again turn toward the light.

Again we see that green plants grow toward sunlight.

How does water rise to the top of plants and trees?

Materials:

A large freshly-cut stalk of celery

A drinking glass

Water

A few drops of ink to color the water

Procedure:

Put the freshly-cut celery stalk into the glassful of colored water.

After a few hours, note that the leaves are colored by the water that has risen through the stalk by capillary action.

Cut the stem crosswise in several places and you will see the tubes that carried the water to the leaves.

Do shoots exert pressure upward?

Materials:

A container of earth

6 beans

24 toothpicks

Pennies

Procedure:

Fill a planting box three-quarters full of earth.

Make it moist but not wet.

Soak six beans in water for six hours.

Shallow plant them equally apart from one another.

Put four toothpicks around each bean so that the penny or pennies can fit inside.

Keep soil moist but not wet and put in the sun.

Watch beans push up one or two or even three pennies.

How can you prove that roots always grow downward and shoots upward?

Materials:

A medium sized jar

Some absorbent cotton

Seeds, such as pumpkin, lima bean, corn or pea

Procedure:

Fill the jar with cotton.

Place the seeds between the cotton and the side of the jar.

Do not place the seeds too close to each other.

Wet the cotton and keep it damp for several days.

After several days, the shoots or stems will be growing upward and the roots will be growing downward.

Invert the glass.

After several more days, the stems and roots will turn so that again the stems grow up and the roots grow down.

If the seeds continue growing in the glass for several days, you will notice that they appear to be dying. Why do you think this happens? The plants seem to be getting everything they need for making their own food—air, water, and sunlight. But they are missing minerals that are found in soil. Up to this point, each plant was living off itself. It was getting nourishment from the food stored in the seed. Now that the plant is ready to make its own food, it needs these minerals.

You can revive the plants by placing them in flowerpots with soil.

5. Do all living things need food and water?

Study the food needs of animals using books, pictures, trips, film.

Study the food needs of plants.

Compare the food needs of plants and animals with the food needs of children.

6. How do we keep food fresh?

Discuss with the children the use of their home refrigerator.

Discuss with the children the use of their home freezer, if they have one.

After a trip to the supermarket or the ice cream store, talk about the use of the freezer to keep foods fresh.

You might point out to the children that there are other ways of keeping foods fresh such as drying foods, canning foods, smoking foods, salting foods and freeze-drying foods.

An older group of children might visit a place like Mount Vernon, where they could see how foods were dried or smoked before refrigeration in order to keep them fresh.

Children are familiar with canned foods since many of their foods come from cans.

   a. You might explain how the food to be canned and the can itself must be heated enough to kill any germs which might cause the food to spoil.
   b. The can must be air tight so that the germs from the air cannot get into the can and spoil the food.

Ask the children how they might keep food cold if they didn't have a refrigerator.

   a. With a little bit of questioning, you might be able to introduce the ice box and the job of the ice man.
   b. The cold cellar could be another topic for discussion on the subject.
   c. Ask the children how a cold running stream could help keep the food fresh on a camping trip. In days past, food was kept cold this way by digging a hole in the ground or building an underground room near a running stream or river.

Growing Things
in the Classroom

(or outside, if possible)

1. Introducing children to the plant world.

Give the children lima beans which have been soaked for about a day and let them discover the little plants inside.

Pass around an avocado seed after opening and tasting the avocado.

Set the avocado seed, pointed end down, in a glass jar filled with water and supported by three toothpicks. Talk with the children about what is happening as you notice together that:

    a. the seed covering has come off.

    b. the top has split and a small plant can be seen inside the crack.

    c. roots appear from the bottom of the seed, one or two at first and then many as time goes on.

Read such books as "The Flower" by Mary Louise Downer and "The Carrot Seed" by Ruth Krauss.

Do finger games and role playing games or songs about digging a garden, including everything a garden needs to grow: sun, rain, earth and air.

Have the children make a poster to place over the classroom plant area showing everything plants need to grow.

Prepare a flannel board* sequential story following the development of a plant from a seed. Have the children tell the story using the flannel board.

2. Learning about fruit plants.

As the children have experiences with and explore different fruits, save the seeds of these fruits and plant them so that the children can begin to appreciate:

    a. that all living things perpetuate themselves.

---

*Fasten a piece of cotton flannel fabric to a stiff board such as poster board. Use felt or felt-backed pieces on the flannel board.

b. that there is life in the things they eat and that all living things are connected in a chain of life.

Orange, lemon, lime, grapefruit and tangerine seeds grow into lovely plants:

a. Plant them immediately after removing them from the fruit or soak them for about 24 hours before planting; in fact, soaking them is a good idea in any case.

b. Add a handful of sand to good potting soil and plant the seeds about 1/2" deep.

c. While germinating seeds, you might cover plants with a plastic meat tray or plastic wrap in order to create a greenhouse effect; a few holes will allow air in.

d. Keep moist on a daily basis but water about twice a week.

The following fruits make good plants:

a. *Pineapple*—Cut off the leafy top and about one inch of the fruit.

You may plant in a shallow pot because the roots do not grow deeply.

Mix gravel or sand in with the soil.

Plant the fruit up to the bottom of the crown.

Pour the water on the leaves so that it will run into the cups at the bottom of the leaves; these cups should be kept full of water.

b. *Avocado*—Place the seed in a jar with water as soon as you remove it from the fruit.

The bottom half of the seed should be in the water, the top half out of the water supported by toothpicks. Do not allow the seed to dry out.

The seed may be planted in soil as well but then the children cannot see the development of the plant from seed.

Germination takes about 30 days.

When the plant has a few leaves, it should be transplanted into soil.

Plant the seed with top half exposed above the soil; be very careful not to damage the roots while transplanting.

Use a pot about 4 inches in diameter.

Mix good potting soil with a little sand and some peat.

3. Learning about vegetable plants.

Introduce the children to the fact that some of the vegetables we eat are not leaves (lettuce) or the fruits (tomato) of the plants, but the roots, such as potatoes, carrots, beets, turnips.

Cultivate some of these roots and tubers and the children will be able to see the relationship of the root they eat to the plant.

The following vegetables make good plants:

a. *Carrot foliage*—Cut off the top end of a carrot and hollow out its center, so as to leave only a thin shell.

Trim the top clean of greenery.

Hang the carrot upside down by pushing 2 toothpicks through the carrot and suspending in a narrow glass of water.

Keep the carrot filled with water and in a short time foliage will start to grow from the bottom upwards toward the light.

b. *Dish plants*—This is another way to "plant" a carrot.

First cut off the leaves on top.

Then cut off about 2 inches of the large end of a carrot. Put this 2 inch piece, top side up, in a shallow dish or bowl.

Put pebbles around it to hold it in place in a standing position.

Keep the pebbles moist and new feathery leaves will start to grow out of the carrot's top.

You can plant the tops of beets in this same way and they will grow green and purple leaves.

You can also plant the tops of radishes and turnips.

c. *Sweet potato vine*—Use a sweet potato that has a few "whiskers".

Put it in a jar of water with its narrow end down.

If you have one, use a jar with an opening that will support the potato.

If not, stick several toothpicks into the thick end of the potato.

Put the jar in a warm, dark place and keep it well filled with water.

New roots will start to grow and, in about 10 days, the stem will start to grow.

As soon as this happens put the jar in a sunny window. Before long, the vine will be full of green foliage.

Beets and onions will send out green leaves and shoots also.

Vegetable seeds to plant:

a. Plant green bean seeds in good potting soil, thin out and keep only the strong plants.

When plants get tall, support by means of string and tape to a window.

If kept watered, you should get string beans.

b. Plant tomato seeds and peas following the directions on the package.

4. What to use for potting and planting.

Besides commercial planters and flower pots, you could use:

a. styrofoam cups which allow you to punch holes in the bottom for drainage.

b. the bottom halves of milk cartons.

c. aluminum baking pans.

Make a window box:

a. Cut away one side of a milk carton and paint the part that is left with poster paints or house paint.

b. Then use the box to hold potted plants or partly fill them with soil and plant flowers and other seeds in them.

157

Make egg flower bowls:

a. To make the opening, tap the side of an egg lightly on a water faucet and then carefully pick the shell from the tapped area.

b. Empty the shell and save the egg for cooking; wash the shell out and turn it upside down to dry.

c. Color the shell in pastel shades of enamel, applying two coats.

d. Then fill the shell with sand or soil and "plant" live, dried or artificial flowers and plants.

e. Plant grass in the shell and paint a face on the shell.

f. The grass then looks like hair.

Make bottle gardens:

a. To make a bottle garden, use a good-sized bottle or jar which has a wide mouth.

b. Put it on the table on its side and put in a layer of pebbles and sand.

c. Cover this foundation with good earth from the back yard.

d. Wet the sand and earth before putting them in the bottle.

e. Now plant your garden, putting the seeds into the bottle on the end of a flat, smooth stick, such as a tongue depressor.

f. Put grass seed in first, to make a green lawn.

g. Then plant some orange, lemon, grapefruit or apple seeds which will grow into little trees or bushes.

h. Next put in some flower seeds of any kind or elm or maple seedlings.

i. Plant a small piece of horseradish root to grow into a hedge.

j. Water your garden sparingly, taking care not to soak the earth since that would rot the seeds. You can use an eyedropper or an atomizer perfume sprayer.

k. Punch several holes in the jar top and screw it in place.

l. This gives the plants air, but you may sometimes have to put a cover on with no holes in it to prevent evaporation.

Make bottle bouquets:

a. This is a method of preserving flowers and leaves in water.

b. Use any flowers you like and make a bouquet of them by adding some sprays of green, such as cosmos leaves or asparagus fern. You can make endless combinations.

c. Tie the stems together with thread and tie the ends of the thread around a stone. Submerge in glass container filled with water.

5. Care of other living things

Make a milk carton bird feeder:

a. Use a 1 or 2 quart milk carton, cutting off the upper part so as to leave the bottom 4 inches high.

b. Slit the four corners down for one inch from the top and bend back the four flaps so the birds can perch on them.

c. Paint the carton green or brown, making holes at each corner for wire or string and hang the feeder from a tree branch.

d. Foods to put in the feeder include bread crumbs, popcorn, rolled oats, raisins, small seed mixtures, corn meal and bits of apples and other fresh and dried fruits.

Make a toilet paper roll or pine cone bird feeder:

a. Prepare a mixture of peanut butter and corn starch.

b. Cover the toilet paper role or pine cone with the mixture.

c. Roll in bird seed.

d. Hang by a string to a tree.

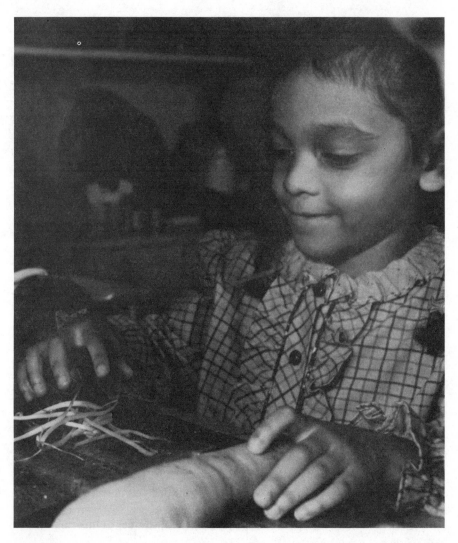

Social Studies
Through Food

1. There are many fruits, vegetables, baked goods, and food preparations which are representative of American ethnic groups or other countries.

2. Encourage the children to share food experiences from their own backgrounds:

   Invite the parents and grandparents of the children to bring to school food from their own home backgrounds for the class to talk about and taste.

   If the parents are unable to come to school during school hours have the children bring in special foods from home.

   The teacher should:

   a. become familiar beforehand with the food to be introduced by either parent or child.

   b. prepare a story of some pictures related to the food or to the culture as a follow-up activity.

   c. encourage the children to discuss with parents, grandparents or others what kinds of foods they ate when they were children and where the foods came from.

3. Introduce foods from around the world:

   Bring to school foods such as mangos, tortillas, pomegranates, etc., and discuss with the children where these foods come from.

   a. Use the Dairy Council picture of children from around the world.

   b. Use a globe.

   c. Use film and filmstrips, if possible.

   d. Learn songs and dances.

   e. Dolls and other representative articles of a culture or country may be used as part of a classroom exhibit.

   f. Invite to school people who come from or lived in other parts of the world.

   g. Embassies and consulates may be excellent sources of information.

Taking Trips
with a School Class

1. Planning a trip

a. Think seriously about whether or not the trip you are planning is valuable and enriching enough to the children and to the program to be worth the time, effort and risk involved.

b. Make sure your goals are clear and will be met.
If possible, visit the place to which you are planning to take the children and speak directly to the person who will be in charge of your visit.
Make sure this person understands how old the children are and is prepared to present the material in a manner relevant to the age of the children.

c. Depending on the age of the children, use good judgment as to the travel time involved.
No trip is worth keeping three-year-old children in cars 45 minutes to an hour one way.

d. If cars are used, make sure the drivers are dependable and there is another adult in the car.

2. Preparing for the trip.

a. Prepare the children for the trip by telling them about it in advance and then having a discussion about the subject, reading a book, seeing a film, etc.

b. Have the children help by decorating their own name and address tags and explain to them how important it is that they wear them.

c. Make sure that the children all have permission slips for the trip from parents or guardians.

d. Find out what the parent's wishes are regarding car seating and use of seat belts.

3. During the trip.

a. Assign an adult to each child; color coding of identification tags might help in setting up groups.

It should be perfectly clear to each adult and to each child which group they belong in and will remain with until they return to the classroom.

b. Groups should be kept small; the ratio of adults to children should be reasonable enough to ensure that the adult has complete control.

c. Use good judgment as to the length of the stay; the children should leave still enthusiastic and interested.

d. Help the children focus and verbalize the experience while it is happening.

4. Follow up.

a. Present activities which help the children remember and sum up their experience.

b. Do not follow up immediately after returning from the trip; allow the children to digest the experience first.

c. Experience charts, dramatic plays, songs, flannel board activities, games and records are just some of the possibilities for follow up activities.

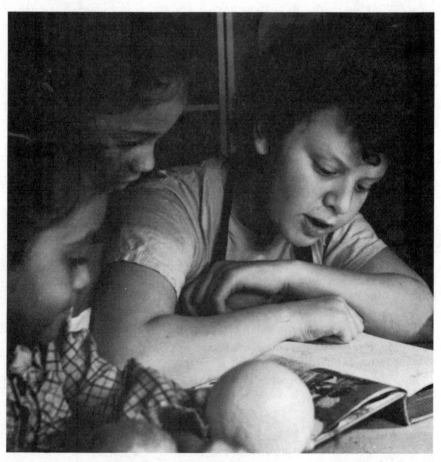

Field Trip Suggestions

Local family farms—Try friends, relatives or acquaintances, or Land Grant Colleges with demonstration farms; ask the local extension agent.

Dairy farms—Local extension agent or local Dairy Council should be of assistance. Milk processing plants or cheese factories should be considered. Try going on a trip to the milk supplier for school or day care center.

Fruit farm or orchard—In some areas growers have opened their fields to public picking from strawberries in late spring to apples before the winter frost. Fruits or vegetables usually available under these arrangments are strawberries, blackberries, raspberries, blueberries, peaches, pears, plums, apples, cherries, tomatoes, beans, squash and potatoes. The cost is considerably lower than those sold in local supermarkets. Consider the excitement of discovery of where produce comes from; the pride in selecting and picking your own makes this adventure one to remember. The Department of Agriculture at the state university may be able to supply you with a list of pick-your-own produce places and approximate harvest dates for each crop. You may want to see the fruit farms at bloom time as well as harvest time.

Corn, wheat, or other grain fields—Good times to visit are planting, growing and harvest times.

Pumpkin patches—Have the children go to pick a pumpkin for Halloween.

Local gardens—Great for those with limited time, budget, and transportation. A neighborhood garden has much to offer at different times during the growing season. Check out the varieties grown, and how plants look as they grow. Can you find the potatoes?

Model farms—Land Grant Colleges may have tours of farms available to children.

Restored villages—May have a general store, flour mills, bakeries, etc.

Grist mills—The local park service may have information.

Local bakery—Check bread wrappers in natural food stores for ideas.

Food market—Try one with a wide variety of stalls, and produce sold directly by the farmer.

Local produce stand—For a mini adventure, try a nearby produce stand and discover what is grown locally.

Cooperative store or local supermarket—See "To Market, To Market", page 124.

Natural food store—Check out varieties of grains and legumes, produce, and protein foods.

Nut store—Check the yellow pages for a listing of such stores.

School food factory—Try a trip to a food depot where food is assembled for satellite feeding.

Cheese plant and milk processing plant—Local Dairy Association may have tours available.

Ethnic food store—Check yellow pages for listings. Compare foods with what is available in the supermarket. Identify the unique foods.

Bon Voyage!

V. SOURCES
AND RESOURCES

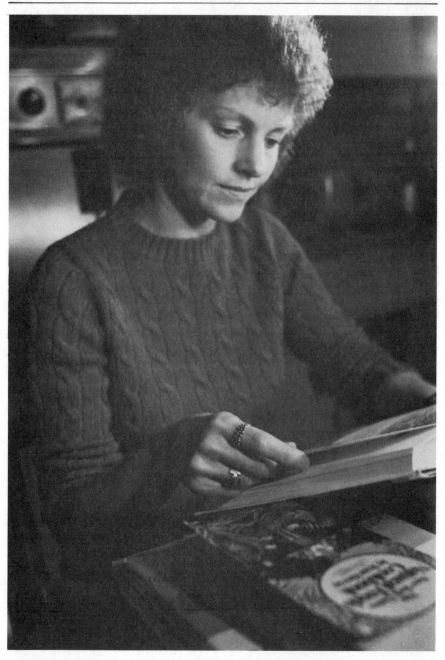

Teacher's Note:

When reading to children, be expressive in voice, face and gesture. Use the book to stimulate discussion. Emphasize references to food. Talk about the variety of foods needed for good health. Help the children compare the ways in which marketing and food preparation have changed over the years, if the book lends itself to such a discussion. Help them notice which foods people eat and which foods animals eat. Point out how families or friends eat together. Mention that food should be returned to the refrigerator to keep it fresh. Reinforce new and descriptive vocabulary. Plan cooking or role-playing activities around the reading of a book.

Books for Children
To Be Used in
Conjunction with
Learning Activities

Vegetables and Fruits

The Great Big Enormous Turnip, Alexes Tolstoy, Franklin Watts, Inc., New York, 1968

The Carrot Seed, Ruth Strauss, Scholastic Book Service, New York, 1971

Stone Soup, Marcia Brown, Charles Scribner, New York, 1947

Pumpkin Moonshine, Tasha Tudor, Henry Z. Walch, Inc., New York, 1962

The Tomato Patch, William Wondriska, Holt, Rhinehart and Winston, New York

The Carrot and Other Root Vegetables, Millicent Selsam, William Morrow, New York, 1970

The Tale of Peter Rabbit, Beatrix Potter, F. Warne & Co., London, 1903

Seeds and More Seeds, Millicent Selsam, Harper & Row, New York, 1959

Partouche Plants a Seed, Ben Schecter, Harper & Row, New York, 1966

Cabbage Moon, Jan Wahl, Holt, Rinehart & Winston, New York, 1965

Bread and Jam for Francis, Russel Hoben, Harper and Row, New York, 1964

A Tree is a Plant, Clyde Bulla, T.Y. Crowell, 1960

The Very Hungry Caterpillar, Eric Carle, Collins-World, 1961

Little Bear (Birthday Soup), Elsa Holmelund Miverick, Harper & Row, New York, 1961

From Seed to Jack O'Lantern, Hannah Johnson, Lothrop, 1978

The Amazing Dandelion, Millicent Selsam and Jerome Wexler, Morrow, 1977

The Story of Johnny Appleseed, Aliki, Prentice Hall, New Jersey, 1963

A Apple Pie, Kate Greenway, Frederick Warne Co., London

Blueberries for Sal, Robert McCloskey, Viking Press, New York, 1966

Buttons and The Magic Apples, W.L. Jenkins Church Kindergarten Resource Book; Josephine Newberry: John Knox Press, Richmond, Va. 1960

Protein

Green Grass and White Milk, Aliki, Thomas Y. Crowell, New York, 1974

The Eggs, Alika, Pantheon Books, New York, 1969

Some Cheese for Charles, Helen Buckley, Lothrop, Lee & Shepard Co., New York, 1963

My Friend the Cow, Lois Lenski, National Dairy Council, Chicago, 1975

Swimmy, Leo Lionni, Pantheon Books, New York, 1963

The Egg Tree, Katherine Milhous, Charles Scribner's Sons, New York, 1950

The Tale of Squirrel Nutkin, Beatrix Potter, Frederick Warne & Co., New York, 1913

One Fish, Two Fish, Red Fish, Blue Fish, Dr. Seuss, Random House, New York, 1960

Scrambled Eggs Super!, Dr. Seuss, Random House, New York, 1953

Pumpkinseeds, Steven Yezback, The Bobbs-Merrill Co., Inc., New York, 1969

Sunflowers for Tina, Anne Norris Baldwin, Four Winds Press, New York, 1970

How Chicks Are Born, Bruce Grant, Rand McNally & Co., Chicago, 1967

The Fisherman And His Boat, Louise Floethe, Charles Scribner's Sons, New York, 1961

The Egg, Dick Bruna, Metheun, 1975

Cereal and Bread

Mr. Picklepaw's Popcorn, Ruth Adams, Lothrop, Lee & Shepard Co., Inc., New York, 1965

Too Many Crackers, Helen Buckley, Lothrop, Lee & Shepard Co., Inc., New York, 1966

Pancakes, Pancakes, Eric Carle, Alfred A. Knopf, New York, 1970

Walter the Baker, Eric Carle, Alfred A. Knopf, Inc., New York, 1972

Squash Pie, Gage Wilson, William Morrow & Company, Inc., New York, 1976

Little Bear's Pancake Party, Janice Berenstein, Lothrop, Lee & Shepard Co., Inc., New York, 1966

The Perfect Pancake, Virginia Kahl, Scribner's Sons, New York, 1960

A Flying Saucer Full of Spaghetti, Fernando Krahn, E.P. Dutton & Co., New York, 1970

"Rice Pudding" *When We Were Very Young,* A.A. Milne, E.P. Dutton & Co., Inc., New York, 1924

Journey Cake Ho!, Ruth Sawyer, The Viking Press, New York, 1953

Chicken Soup With Rice, Maurice Sendak, Harper & Row, New York, 1962

The Little Red Hen, The Golden Press, New York

The Rolling Rice Ball, Junichi Yoda, Parents' Magazine Press, New York, 1969

Boy the Baker, The Miller and More, Harold Benson, Crown Books, 1975

Other

The Big Honey Hunt, Janice and Stanley Berenstein, Beginner Books, Random House, New York, 1962

Watch Honeybees With Me, Judy Hawes, Thomas Y. Crowell, New York 1964

General

A Tree Is Nice, Janice May Udry, Harper & Brothers, New York, 1956

Have You Seen Trees, Joanne Oppenhein, Addison-Wesley Publishing Co., Reading, Mass. 1967

I'm A Big Helper, Sylvia Tester, David C. Cook Publishing Co., Elgin, Ill., 1963

The Man Who Didn't Wash His Dishes, Phyllis Krasilovsky, Doubleday & Co., Jr. Books, Garden City, New York, 1950

Let's Play House, Lois Lenski, Henry Z. Walck, Inc., New York

My Color Game, Evelyn M. Begley, Whitman Tell-A-Tale Book, Whitman Publishing Co., Inc., Racine, Wisconsin, 1966

I See Something Red, Elisa Scott, Hallmark Children's Edition, Kansas City, Mo.

Hailstones and Halibut Bones, Mary O'Neill, Doubleday & Co., Inc., Garden City, New York, 1961

Mother Goose Nursery Rhymes

A Child's Garden of Verses, Robert Louis Stevenson

Nursery Tales:
    The Gingerbread Boy
    The Three Bears
    Jack and The Beanstalk
    Three Billy Goats Gruff
    The Little Red Hen

The Flower, Mary Louise Downer, Will R. Scott Inc., New York, 1955

What Shall I Put In The Hole That I Dig?, Eleanor Thompson, Whitman Tell-A-Tale Book, Western Publishing Co., Racine, Wisconsin

Once We Went on a Picnic, Aileen Fisher, T.Y. Crowell, 1975

The Plant Sitter, Gene Zion, Harper & Row Publishers, New York, 1959

A Day On The Farm, Nancy Fielding Hulick, Golden Press, New York, 1960

Come To The Farm, Ruth Tensen, Reilly & Lee Co., Publishers, Chicago, 1949

Autumn Harvest, Alvan Tresselt, Lothrop, 1951

Wake Up Farm, Alvan Tresselt, Lothrop, 1955

The Little Farm, Lois Lenski, Henry Z. Walck, Inc., New York, 1942

Big Red Barn, Margaret Wise Brown, Addison-Wesley Publishing Co., Reading, Mass., 1965

Hard Scrabble Harvest, Dahlow Ipcar, Doubleday, 1976

To Market To Market, Emma L. Brock, Alfred A. Knopf, New York, 1930

Books Which Can Be Used by the Teacher with Younger Children or Read by Older Children

Milk For You, G. Warren Schloat, Charles Scribner Sons, New York, 1951

Animals That Give People Milk, Terrance W. McCabe & Harley W. Mitchell, National Dairy Council, Chicago, Illinois, 1970

The Wonderful Egg, G. Warren Schloat, Charles Scribner Sons, New York, 1952

Plants That Feed Us, Carroll Lane Fenton & Hermine B. Kitchen, John Day & Co., New York 1971 (the story of grains and vegetables)

Foxfire Books, Eliot Wigginton, Doubleday & Co., Garden City, New York

Growing Up, How We Become Alive, Are Born and Grow, Karl de Schweinitz, MacMillan Co., New York, 1965

The Secret World of the Baby, Beth Day and Margaret Liley, M.D., Random House, New York, 1968

The Little House in the Big Woods, Laura Ingalls Wilder, Harper & Row, New York, 1953

The Little House on the Prairie, Laura Ingalls Wilder, Harper and Row, New York, 1953

Grains, Elizabeth B. Brown, Prentice Hall, 1977 (history of grain)

Popcorn, Millicent E. Selsam, Morrow, 1976 (history of maize)

Hunters Stew and Hangtown Fry, Lila Perl, (what colonial America ate), Seabury Press, 1977

The Bakery Factory, Aylette Jenness, T. Crowell, 1978

Wild Foods, Lawrence Pringle, Scribner, 1978

Good For Me: All About Food in 32 Bites, Marilyn Burns, Little Company, 1978

Fruits We Eat, Carroll Lane Fenton and Hermine B. Kitchen, John Day Co., New York, 1961

Plants In the City, Herman and Nina Schneider, (a good handbook to help introduce plants to children) John Day Co., New York, 1951

The First Book of Food, Ida Scheib, Franklin Watts Publishers, New York, 1956

The Carrot and Other Root Vegetables, Millicent E. Selsam, William Morrow & Co., New York, 1970

We Read About Seeds And How They Grow, Harold E. Tannenbaum and Nathan Sillman, Webster Publishing Co., St. Louis, Missouri, 1960

The Tomato And Other Fruit Vegetables, Millicent E. Selsam, William Morrow & Co., New York, 1970

Eating And Cooking Around The World, Erick Barry, John Day Co., New York, 1963

Plants That Feed The World, Rose E. Frisch, D. Van Nostrand Co., Princeton, New Jersey, 1966

The Wonderful World of Food, John Boyd Orr, Garden City Books, New York, 1958

Plants Are Like That, A. Harris Stone and Peter Plascencia, (a chemistry book about plants for young children) Prentice-Hall, Englewood Cliffs, New Jersey, 1968

The Chemistry Of A Lemon, A. Harris Stone and Peter Plascencia, (exciting experiments with lemons) Prentice-Hall Inc., Englewood Cliffs, New Jersey, 1966

Salt, Augusta Golden, (good experiments for preschool and early primary) Thomas Crowell Co., New York, 1965

The First American Peanut Growing Book, Kathy Mandry, Random House, 1976

Apple Orchard, Irmengarde Eberle, Henry Z. Walck Inc., New York, 1962

And Everything Nice, Eliza K. Cooper (the story of sugar, spice and flavorings) Harcourt Brace and World Inc., New York, 1966

Rice, Food For a Hungry World, Winnefred Hammond, Coward McCann, Inc., 1961

Nothing To Eat But Food, Frank Jupo, (a history of food for young children) E.P. Dutton and Co., Inc., New York, 1954

Measure With Metric, Franklyn Branley, T. Crowell, 1975

The First Book of Gardening, Virginia Kirkus, Franklin Watts Inc., New York, 1956

The Indoor Outdoor Grow It Book, S. Sinclair Baker, Random House, New York, 1966

Indoor Outdoor Gardening Book, Cynthia and Alvin Koehler, Grosset & Dunlap, Inc. (Wonder Books), New York, 1969

A Gardening Book: Indoors and Outdoors, Anne B. Walsh, Athenum, 1976

Kids Gardening: First Indoor Outdoor Gardening Book For Children, Aileen Paul, Doubleday, 1972

Books with Background Material for the Teacher

Science Experiences for the Early Childhood Years, Jean Durgin Harlan, Charles E. Merrill Co., Columbus, Ohio, 1976.

Beginnings, Teacher's Guide Science Curriculum Improvement Study, Rand McNally and Company, Chicago, Illinois, 1974

The Organic Living Book, Bernice Kohn, Viking Press, New York, 1972

Good Earth Almanac, 2210 West 75 Street, Suite 305, Prairie Village, Kansas, 66208

Farming In The Classroom—Teachers' Guide, Science Study Aid No. 8, Agricultural Research Service, U.S. Department of Agriculture, Supt. of Documents, Government Printing Office, Washington, D.C.

Gardening In Containers—A Handbook, Brooklyn Botanical Gardens, Brooklyn, N.Y.

Food in History, Reay Tannahill, Stein and Day Publishers, New York, 1973

How Do Your Children Grow?, Association For Childhood Education International, 3615 Wisconsin Avenue, N.W., Washington, D.C. 20016

Nutrition And Intellectual Growth in Children, Association For Childhood Education International, 3615 Wisconsin Avenue, N.W., Washington, D.C. 20016

Food Selection For Good Nutrition In Group Feeding, Agricultural Research Service, Dept. of Agriculture, Supt. of Documents, U.S. Government Printing Office, Washington, D.C.

Selection and Care of Fresh Fruits and Vegetables, 1977, United Fresh Fruit & Vegetable Association, 1019 19th Street, N.W., Washington, D.C. 20036

Let's Go Metric (Chapter 7), Frank Donovan, Weybright and Talley, 1974

Cookbooks

The Story Cookbook, Carol MacGregor, Doubleday & Co., Inc., New York, 1959

Love At First Bite, Jane Cooper, Alfred Knopf, Inc., 1977

The Cook Book of Breads, Sunset Lane Books, Menlo Park, California, 1973

The Down To Earth Cookbook, Anita Borghese, Charles Scribner and Sons, New York, 1973

The Mother Child Cook Book, Nancy Ferrerra, Pacific Coast Publishing Co., Menlo Park, California 94025

The Lucky Cookbook For Boys and Girls, (easy to read and easy to cook), Eva Moore Talwaldis, Scholastic Book Services, 1972

Kids Are Natural Cooks; Child Tested Recipes For Home and School Using Natural Foods, Guidelines for Teachers and Parents by the Parents' Nursery School, Cambridge, Mass., 02138

The Good For Me Cookbook, (Ages 3-12), Karen B. Croft, Rand E. Research Associates, San Francisco, California, 1971 (Order from: Karen B. Croft, 741 Maplewood Place, Palo Alto, California 94303)

Science Experiments You Can Eat, Vicki Cohl, J.B. Lippincott Co., Philadelphia, 1973

Cooking and Eating With Children, Oralie McAfee, Evelyn W. Haines and Barbara B. Young, Association for Childhood Education International, Washington, D.C. 1974

Cool Cooking for Kids, Pat McClenahan and Ida Jaqua, Fearon Publishers, Inc., Belmont, California, 1976

Kids Kitchen Takeover, Sara Stein, 1977

Laurel's Kitchen, L. Robertson and C. Flenders and B. Godfrey, Nilgiri Press, Berkeley, California, 1977

The Moosewood Cookbook, M. Katzen (Vegetable Cookbook); Ten Speed Press, P.O. Box 7123, Berkeley, California 94707

Many Hands Cooking: An International Cookbook for Girls and Boys, Terry T. Cooper and Marilyn Ratner, T. Crowell Company (in cooperation with the United States Committee for UNICEF), 1974

Music Books,
Records, Films and
Suggestions

Songbooks

Songs For Children, A Whitman Book, Western Publishing Co., Inc., Racine, Wisconsin

Singing Fun, Lucille F. Wood and Louise B. Scott, Webster Division, McGraw Hill Co., New York, 1954

Heritage Songster, Leon and Lynn Dallin, William C. Brown Company, Dubuque, Iowa, 1966

This is Music for Today, Kindergarten and Nursery School, Adeline McCall, Allyn and Bacon, Inc., 1971

The Fireside Book of Children's Songs, Marie Winn (editor), Simon and Schuster, New York, 1956

Records and Songs to Sing:

In My Garden, words and music by Jeremy and Alan Arkin, "Songs and Fun With The Baby Sitters", Vangard Records, VRS 9053

What Food Should We Eat Every Day, Now We Know Series with Tom Glazer and Paul Tripp, Columbia Records CL 670

How Does A Cow Make Milk?, Now We Know Series with Tom Glazer and Paul Tripp, Columbia Records CL 670

Record Set For All Seasons, Bowmar Catalogue, Glendale, California, CRG records

The following records are Childrens Record Guild (CRG) records, New York, William P. Scott, Inc., Publisher. Division of the American Recording Society.

1. *I'm Dressing Myself,* Philip List. CRG #1-803A
2. *Every Day We Grow 1-0,* Tom Glazer CRG #8001/2 A-d (two records)
3. *The Carrot Seed* as told by Norman Rose CRG #1003 A-B

Suggestions

Use your imagination and make up food and planting songs and action games using such familiar tunes and games as:

Paw Paw Patch	*Twinkle, Twinkle Little Star*
Simon Says	*Aiken Drum*
Mulberry Bush	*Put Your Finger In The Air*
Old MacDonald Had A Farm	*London Bridge*
Row, Row, Row Your Boat	*Etc., etc., etc.*

Creative Dramatics

Creative Movement for the Developing Child, Clare Cherry, Fearon Publishers, Belmont, California, 1971

Journal of Creative Behavior, 7 (First Quarter, 1973), 37-53; "Let's Be An Ice Cream Machine!". Gary A. Davis, Charles J. Helfert and Gloria R. Shapiro.

Fingerplays

Let's Do Fingerplays, Marion F. Grayson, Robert B. Luce, Inc., Washington, D.C. 1962

For Film and Filmstrip Information, Refer to:

Your local public library: Film Service Catalogue and Supplements. Refer to the following categories:

Nutrition
Health
Vitamins and Minerals
Cooking
Obesity

See the following sections in the catalogue:

Children's Films
Children's Poetry
Children's Stories

American Library Association Film catalogues, 50 East Huron Street, Chicago, Illinois, 60611

More Films Kids Love, Maureen Gaffney, 1977

Guide to Educational Media: Films, Filmstrips, Multimedia Kits, Programmed Instruction Materials, Recordings, Slides, Transparencies, Videotapes, Margaret Rufsvold

Multimedia Approach to Children's Literature, E. Green and M. Schoenfeld (a selective list of films, filmstrips and recordings based on children's books)

Educational Film Library Association, 43 West 61 Street, New York, N.Y. 10023 (212) 246-4533

Modern Talking Picture Service, 2000 L Street, N.W., Washington, D.C.

Weston Woods Catalogue, Weston, Connecticut 06880

Teaching Resources Films, 83 East Avenue, Norwalk, Connecticut 06851
  1. *The Little Red Hen*
  2. *Nail Soup*
  3. *The Story of Johnny Appleseed*

The National Apple Month, Inc., 2430 Pennsylvania Avenue, N.W., Washington, D.C. 20034
  The Story of How Apples Grow, a filmstrip, plus other films, filmstrips and books

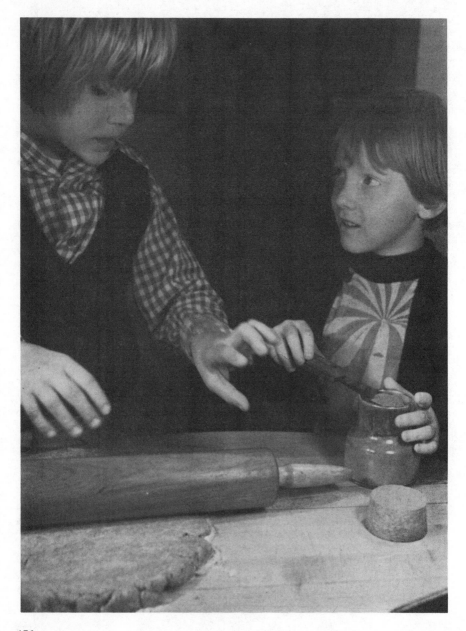

Other Materials and Useful Addresses

David C. Cook Publishing Co., Elgin, Illinois 60120
  Teaching Pictures:
  1. Social Studies; A Trip To The Farm
  2. Science; Plants and Seeds
  3. Health; Food and Nutrition; Health and Cleanliness

Scholastic Book Services, New York
  Picture Collection:
  1. Fruit and Vegetables
  2. The Rural Environment

Teaching Resources, 100 Boylston Street, Boston, Massachusetts 02115
  Fruit and Animal Puzzles

Dennison Manufacturing Co., Framingham, Massachusetts
  Bulletin Board Picture Sets:
  1. The Farm
  2. Food
  3. The Family

General Learning Corporation, The Judy Co., 310 North Second Street, Minneapolis, Minnesota 55401
  Judy Puzzles and Judy Story Sets
  Judy See-Quees (Sequence story puzzles)
  1. Brushing Teeth
  2. Grocery Shopping
  3. Story of Milk
  4. Helping Mother

The Milton Bradley Co., Springfield, Massachusetts
  Flannelboard figures:
  1. Farm Animals
  2. The Family
  3. The Seasons

Instructor Publications, Inc., Dansville, N.Y. 14437
  Instructor Primary Science Concept Chart

Rice Council, P.O. Box 22802, Houston, Texas 77027 (Free booklet available)

Florida Citrus Commission, Lakeland, Florida 33802

U.S. Department of Agriculture, Washington, D.C. 20250. Nutrition Charts

Kansas Wheat Commission, 1021 North Main, Hutchinson, Kansas 67501

Green Giant Co., LeSeuer, Minnesota 56058

And don't forget:

The local School System Library or media center
The Health Department
The Heart Association
The University Agricultural Extension Service
Consumer Protection Agencies
Consumer Action Groups

National 4-H Club Foundation, 7100 Connecticut Avenue, Washington, D.C. 20015

The U.S. Committee for UNICEF, (International Cookbooks, food books), 331 East 38th Street, New York, N.Y. 10016

Journal of Nutrition Education, Society of Nutrition Education, 2140 Shattucle Avenue, Suite 111, Berkeley, California 94704

Food and Nutrition Information Center, National Agricultural Library, U.S. Department of Agriculture, Baltimore Blvd., Beltsville, Md.

National Institutes of Health, 9000 Rockville Pike, Bethesda, Md. 20014
Nutrition Coordinating Committee
National Institute of Child Health and Human Development
Public Information Office

Educational Materials Review Center (EDMARC), Office of Education, U.S. Department of Health, Education and Welfare, 400 Maryland Avenue, S.W., Washington, D.C. 20202

Superintendent of Documents, U.S. Government Printing Office, Washington, D.C. 20402

Consumer Information Center, Pueblo, Colorado 81009
Food and nutrition
Health
Gardening
Consumer protection

United Fresh Fruit and Vegetable Association, 727 N. Washington St., Alexandria, Va. 22314

Produce Marketing Associations

Other Fruit, Vegetable and Grain Growers Associations

Center For Science In The Public Interest, 1755 S St., N.W., Washington, D.C. 20009. Send for publications list.

The compilation on the preceeding pages has been prepared in order to bring to the attention of those individuals working with children the rich variety of excellent resources available to meet different group or program needs. We want to thank the Child Development Department, University of Maryland, for sharing the bibliography they prepared so that we could enrich our own bibliography for the Sources and Resources section.

There are pictures and charts prepared by dairy, cereal and other commercial associations and companies, which can be constructively used, such as *We All Like Milk,* produced by the Dairy Council. However, the important guidelines discussed on the following page should be kept in mind.

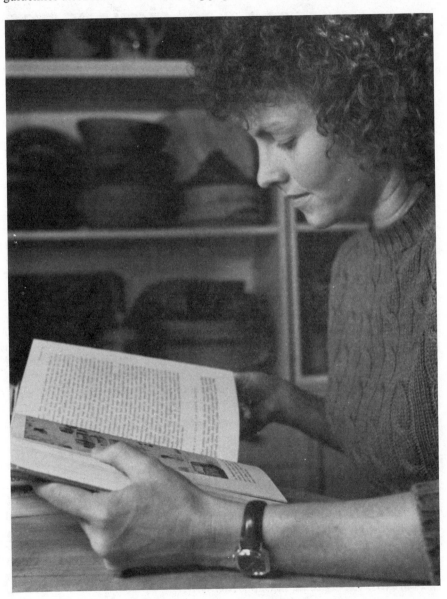

How to Use Nutritional Resources Developed by Special Interest Groups, Food Associations and Food Industries

Nutrition educational materials developed with funds from vested interest groups should be carefully scrutinized to protect the integrity of nutrition knowledge. A food association may put a heavy emphasis on those foods which are products of companies who fund them such as cereal or dairy industries. The educational material promoted may not give the full scope of information about a product, including certain limitations which should be considered. For example, the dairy industry may equate ice cream, one of its products, with milk, even though it doesn't have the same nutrient density as milk. Ice cream is high in sugar and saturated fat, but since most people enjoy it, it should be eaten as a treat on special occasions rather than as a part of the daily food pattern.

Powdered skim milk and fortified margarine make a contribution to our daily food needs. However, one may have difficulty in finding references to these foods in information prepared by certain dairy concerns. Information developed by industries whose products are high in cholesterol or saturated fat may not give a balanced presentation of the role of these dietary components as potential risk factors in heart disease.

The following guidelines may be of some assistance in using resources:
1. What interest groups have produced the materials?
2. Is the information consistent with the promotion of good eating habits?
3. Is there acceptable evidence for the statements made?
4. Is the information presented complete?

Nutrition education is too important to be primarily in the hands of vested interest, mainly interested in selling products rather than in educating the public to make wise food choices. Nutrition education, like any formal education, should be taught by persons such as nutritionists, educators and professionals in related fields, concerned with the public interest rather than by persons involved in promoting a product.

VI. LUNCHES, SNACKS AND CELEBRATIONS

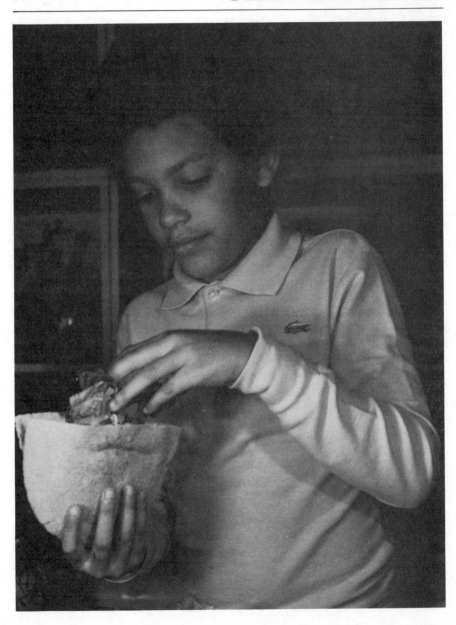

How to Take the "Drag" Out of Bag Lunches

The food children eat affects their learning and behavior, as well as their growth and development. Hungry children have difficulty concentrating on school work and have a tendency to become restless and over-active. The noon meal is very important and should include the following:

1. One half-pint of lowfat milk, skim milk, lowfat yogurt or buttermilk.
2. Two ounces (edible protein as served) of lean meat, poultry, or fish; or 2 ounces of cheese; or one egg; or one-half cup of cooked dry beans or peas; or 4 tablespoons of peanut butter, or an equivalent quantity of any combinations of the above listed foods.
3. A three-fourths cup serving consisting of two or more vegetables or fruits, or both.
4. One slice of whole grain or enriched bread.

Planning Lunches—Good for Picnics, Too!

1. Sandwiches prepared the night before or in the morning before leaving for school should be safe to eat, if properly handled. Proper handling means good sanitation, adequate cooking and refrigeration.
2. If the food was properly handled at home with the sandwiches being chilled or frozen, it should be safe to eat at lunch time at school, even if not refrigerated at school.
3. Sandwiches could be wrapped in foil and frozen the night before. With care, foil may be reused as well as recycled.
4. When freezing sandwiches, omit lettuce or other greens unless chopped with filling. Wrap lettuce or greens separately. Add to sandwiches at time of eating.
5. A small thermos with a wide mouth might be a good investment. It can be used to carry such things as chili, sliced fresh fruit, crispy lettuce, or coleslaw....foods that might add variety to a packed lunch.
6. Try to use leftover meats as sandwich fillers, e.g., chicken salad made from leftover chicken or even a cold chicken leg might be a welcome change.
7. Save small plastic tubs about 6-8 ounce size (soft margarine containers).

The containers are good for carrying salad, puddings and fruit.

8. Children usually find raw vegetables fun to eat. They have more vitamins than when you cook them.
9. Desserts should be kept simple. Try fruit, pumpkin seeds, sunflower seeds, peanuts, raisins, puddings or a plain cookie.
10. Children usually like cheese and crackers for lunch. If possible you could send a small thermos of soup along with them.
11. If you are sending cut fresh fruit such as bananas, apple wedges or peach halves, dip the cut part of the fruit in any type of citrus juice such as lemon, orange or grapefruit juice. This prevents the fruit from turning brown. Dipping fruit in salted water or vinegar will also prevent the fruit from turning brown.
12. A piece of fruit will cost no more and usually less than packaged pies, potato chips, corn chips and other heavily processed foods which too often are included in packed lunches for children.

Sandwich Ideas

Egg: Chop hard-cooked egg and mix with salad dressing. For variety, add one or a combination of the following:

Onion	Bean Sprouts	Chopped Raw Spinach
Celery	Lettuce	Grated Cheese
Raisins	Grated Carrot	Green Pepper
Chicken		

Cheese: Sliced or grated with salad dressing. For variety, add:

Chopped Nuts	Chopped Onion	Crushed Pineapple

Cottage Cheese: For variety, mix with:

Cucumber	Chopped Fruit	Nuts
Tomatoes	Green Pepper	Sliced Banana
Apple Sauce	Caraway Seeds	

Or, spread bread with: Tomato sauce and oregano, brown mustard.

Peanut Butter: Plain or with one of the following:

Raisins	Molasses	Chopped Prunes
Nuts	Sliced Apple	Sliced Banana
Shredded Carrots	Sprouts	

Baked Beans: Plain or mashed with chopped onion and a small amount of chili sauce or raisins.

Hummus: See recipes.

Split Pea Spread: See recipes.

Fish:
Tuna with salad dressing; add chopped celery, peanuts, apple slices or raisins.
White fish with chopped celery, catsup, salad dressing.
Salmon with salad dressing; add chopped celery.
Sardines plain or with salad dressing.

Meat:
Chicken sliced or chopped with salad dressing and shredded raw greens.
Beef sliced or chopped with salad dressing, mustard and shredded raw greens.
Turkey sliced with nuts, celery, pineapple or apple slices.

Breads

Whole grain breads such as whole wheat, rye, cracked wheat are best. If white bread is used, be sure it is enriched. Use loaf bread, flat bread, rolls, muffins, biscuits, tortillas, bagels, quick bread, steamed bread.

Fruits and/or Vegetables (something crisp or juicy)

Raw Vegetables

Carrot Strips	Cauliflower Florets
Celery Sticks	Cucumber Strips
Lettuce Wedges	Kohlrabi Slices
Spinach Leaf	Small Tomato or Wedge
Turnip Sticks	Green Pepper Strips
Endive Pieces	Raw Potato Pieces
Radishes	Cabbage Leaves

Fruits

Apples	Apricots
Bananas	Berries
Cherries	Grapefruit
Grapes	Oranges
Peaches	Pears
Plums	Tangerines
Melon Wedges	Seedless Grapes
Strawberries	Pineapple Wedges, fresh

Nutritious Treats

Raisins	Sunflower
Nuts	Peanut Butter ball rolled in roasted
Granola	sesame seeds
Pumpkin Seeds	

These items may be purchased in large units. A small amount wrapped in a twist of waxed paper could be placed in the lunch bag.

Milk

Lowfat milk, skim milk, lowfat yogurt or buttermilk. Try a milkshake with powdered milk, banana, or orange juice with a dash of cinnamon on top.

Foods to Avoid

Foods which should be avoided are those which contain excessive amounts of saturated fat, sugar or potentially harmful food additives such as in soft drinks, candy, jellied sugar doughnuts, potato chips, corn chips, sticky cakes, cookies and rich pastries. These foods have little or no nutritional value and are usually high in calories and cost.

---

*Canned fruits may be taken in bag lunch if put in tightly covered plastic container. Drain the sugary syrup.

Packed Lunches

White Fish Sandwich with catsup and Parsley
Celery Wagon
Granola
Lowfat Yogurt
Lowfat Milk

Peanut Butter and Banana Sandwich
Carrot Sticks
Hard Cooked Egg
Lowfat Milk

Bean Sandwich on Whole Wheat Bread
Coleslaw or Grated Carrots
Apple
Lowfat Milk

Cottage Cheese and Raisin Sandwich on Boston Brown Bread
Pepper Rings
Orange
Lowfat Milk

Scrambled Egg Sandwich
Fresh Tomato or Spinach Leaves
Pumpkin or Sunflower Seeds
Lowfat Milk

Sliced Turkey, Lettuce and Biscuit Sandwich
Baked Sweet Potato
Green Pepper Strips
Lowfat Milk

Cheddar Cheese and Bean Sprout Sandwich
Banana
Lowfat Milk

Tuna Salad on Roll
Green Pepper and Carrot Sticks
Pear or Plum
Lowfat Milk

Turkey Salad Sandwich
Green Salad
Orange Juice
Milk Pudding
Lowfat Milk

Chopped Egg Sandwich
Orange Wedges
Peanuts
Lowfat Milk

Salmon Salad Sandwich with Lettuce
Carrot Strips or Spinach Leaves
Banana
Lowfat Milk

Swiss Cheese Sandwich with Lettuce on Whole Wheat Bread
Tangerine
Lowfat Milk

Baked Bean and Raw Vegetable
 Sandwich (or Stewed Beans)
Melon or Pineapple Wedge
Lowfat Milk

Cottage Cheese and Pineapple on
 Nut Bread
Cherry Tomatoes
Oatmeal Cookie
Lowfat Milk

Riceburger
Tomatoes
Hard Cooked Egg
Oatmeal Muffin
Lowfat Milk

Chicken Wings or Drumstick
Roll or Muffin with Margarine
Fruit Salad
Peanuts
Lowfat Milk

Chopped Chicken Liver Sandwich
 on Rye Bread
Parsley and Cucumber Fingers
Apple
Lowfat Milk

Tuna Fish and Lettuce Sandwich on
 Whole Wheat Bread
Fresh Tomato or Coleslaw
Lowfat Milk

Surprises

On special occasions, include a favorite treat in the packed lunch. A message like "You Are Magnificent", a short poem, a funny drawing, or a portrait on an open face sandwich. For the face, use peanut butter or cream cheese, carrot curls or parsley for hair, green pepper, apple, nuts and raisins for the eyes and nose. Make a celery wagon with carrot slices on toothpicks for wheels. Put the message inside the wagon.

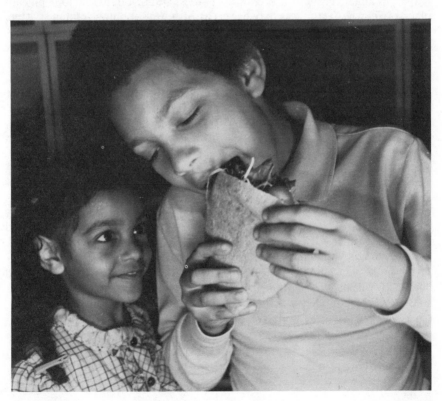

Nutritious Snacks

Vegetable Snacks: Cut up fresh raw vegetables. For example, celery, carrots, cauliflower, broccoli, green pepper, green beans, green peas, cucumber strips, turnip sticks, zucchini. Serve alone or with peanut butter, cottage cheese, cream cheese or ricotta.

Fresh Fruit Snacks: Slice or serve whole: apples, apricots, bananas, berries, grapes, oranges, grapefruit sections, peaches, pears, plums, melon, pineapple, strawberries, etc. Slices may be served with peanut butter, cottage cheese, yogurt, cream cheese, ricotta cheese. Try a new exotic fruit once a week—quince, prickly pear, pomegranate, kiwi, persimmon, kumquats, mangoes, papaya.

Dried Fruit Snacks: Try raisins, apricots, dates, figs, prunes, apples, pears, etc. Dried fruit may be eaten alone or with nuts (peanuts, walnuts, almonds, cashews), or with seeds (sunflower, pumpkin) or unsweetened coconut.

Nuts and Seeds: Pumpkin, sunflower, peanuts, pecans, walnuts, etc. Mix with raisins. *Do not give seeds or nuts to children under four.*

Grain Products:

A. *Whole wheat bread and crackers:* Read the label! Make sure the first ingredient is whole wheat. Try a variety of yeast breads and quick breads—whole wheat, rye, oatmeal, mixed grains, bran—plain or with dried fruit. Try rye crisps, whole grain flat bread, and whole grain crackers. Serve bread and crackers with cheese, peanut butter and sliced bananas (with a dash of honey), and a glass of lowfat milk.

B. *Dry Cereals:* Choose unsweetened varieties. For example: Spoon-sized shredded wheat, 100% bran, grapenuts, 40% bran, homemade granola, toasted wheat germ. Serve plain or with milk. Add dried fruit, nuts and seeds.

C. *Popcorn:* Try using grated cheese (for example, parmesan) instead of salt and butter.

D. *Plain Cookies:* Bake your own cookies, substituting 1/2 whole wheat flour for white flour, or use all whole wheat. Try oatmeal, peanut butter or molasses cookies. Serve cookies with lowfat milk.

E. *Whole Wheat Baked Products:* Avoid rich cakes, pastries, cookies. Instead buy or bake whole wheat muffins and pancakes, bran muffins, corn muffins. Substitute whole wheat flour in your favorite recipes for white flour.

Beverages:

A. Use fruit juices and vegetable juices rather than fruit drinks which are high in sugar and lower in vitamins.

B. *Lowfat Milk:* Serve plain with bread, crackers, cereal, etc. Mix in blender with banana or other fruit, orange juice and ice for a healthy milkshake. Try heating milk with 1 teaspoon vanilla extract (or other favorite extract flavor), plus 1 teaspoon honey or molasses and a dash of cinnamon. Make your own eggnog (the commercial variety is expensive and too sweet). Mix 1 cup milk and 1 raw egg in blender. Add 1/4 teaspoon vanilla, 1 teaspoon honey and a dash of nutmeg. For more variety, try lowfat yogurt and buttermilk. Culture your own.

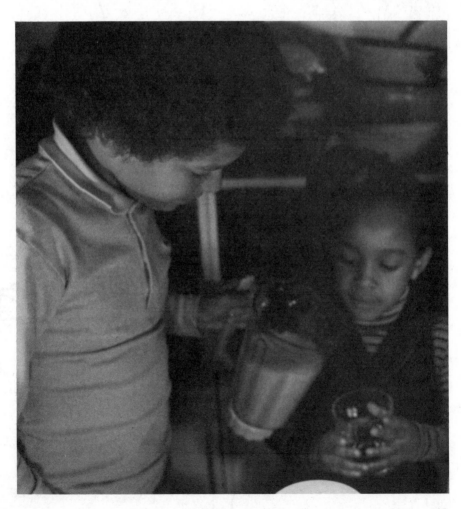

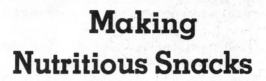

Making Nutritious Snacks

FOR YOUR KIDS—AND FOR YOU, TOO!

Since all kids—and adults, too—eat snacks, serve the best!

Vegetable Snacks:
Tomato, Green Pepper, Cucumber, Zucchini, Green Beans, Mushrooms
Flowers: Raw Broccoli and Cauliflower

Leaves: Cabbage, Lettuce, Parsley, Watercress

Stems: Celery, Green Onions

Roots: Carrots, Radish, Turnip

Serve alone or with: Peanut Butter, Cottage Cheese Yogurt, Cream or Ricotta Cheese

Drinks
Use Fruit Juices and Tomato Juice instead of Fruit Drinks.

Milk: serve plain or blended with Banana or other fruit, Orange Juice and ice for a healthy milkshake.

Try Roasted Soybeans, Too!

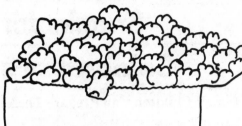

Grain Products

1. *Popcorn*
2. *Buy* Wholegrain Bread and Crackers (not caramel colored)
3. *Baking Your Own* Use flours from whole grains; Yeast Bread Quick Bread, Muffins, Biscuits and Pancakes
4. *Dry Cereals* Choose unsweetened varieties like: Shredded Wheat, 100% Bran, Grapenuts and Homemade Granola

READ THE LABEL!!!!!!

Fresh Fruits Snacks

Apples, Apricots, Bananas, Berries, Cherries, Grapes, Melons, Oranges, Peaches, Plums, Pears, etc.

Slices may be served with peanut butter, Cottage Cheese, Yogurt, Cream or Ricotta Cheese.

If canned fruit, rinse off the syrup.

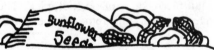

Dried Fruit Snacks:

Try—Raisins, Apricots, Dates, Figs, Prunes, Dried Apples or Pears. *Alone or with* Nuts, Seeds—Sunflower Pumpkin or Unsweetened Coconut

CAUTION:

Children under 4 may choke on Nuts, Seeds, and Popcorn

Snacks for Celebrations

(Small Children Can Prepare These)

Satellite Balls: Select a red apple or an orange. Stick toothpicks with the following tidbits all around the apple or orange:

Pineapple	Grapes	Cheese Cubes

1" long stalks of stuffed celery
Prunes stuffed with Peanut Butter or Part-Skim Ricotta Cheese

Cheese Balls: Combine lowfat cottage cheese or grated cheddar cheese with a little salad dressing, form into small balls, roll in chopped parsley or chopped peanuts.

Stuffed Prunes: Pit prunes, stuff with peanut butter or part-skim ricotta cheese.

Stuffed Celery: One inch long celery ribs stuffed with part-skim riccota cheese or peanut butter.

Fruit Kabobs: Put variety of small pieces of fruit on toothpick. These could be apple wedges, raisins, orange sections, pineapple, grapes, melon balls, prunes.

Vegetable Kabobs: Same as fruit, only use a variety of vegetables such as cherry tomatoes, parsley, carrot circles, pepper squares, turnip triangles.

Apple: Cut apple into small wedges, place on toothpicks with raisins.

Funny Faces: Cut bread in circles with a cookie cutter. Spread with cheese, cottage cheese, peanut butter, and decorate with dots of fruit, vegetables, nuts, or seeds (pumpkin, poppy, sunflower, caraway).

Vegetable Flowers: Cut a peeled turnip into thin slices. With a scalloped-shaped cookie cutter, cut shapes from the slices. Slice a peeled carrot to make carrot circles. Put turnip, then carrot on a toothpick. Use parsley or watercress to make foliage for the carrot-turnip flowers.

Cheese Pumpkins: Soften cheddar cheese, moisten with salad dressing, shape into tiny balls. Roll in paprika. Score with a toothpick at 1/4 inch intervals, flatten at top and bottom. Stick a raisin in the top for a pumpkin stem.

Popcorn and Peanuts are always good additions to a party.

Children's Calendar
of Celebrations

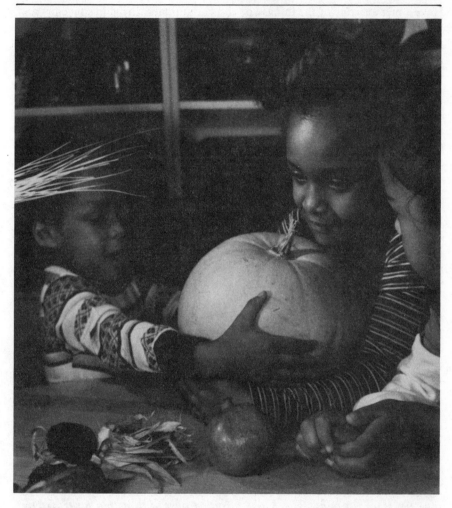

Children need to feel a sense of belonging; to know their roots and ethnic heritage. You may want to make a calendar to celebrate ethnic occasions that are significant to the children. Have them share any special customs and ethnic foods that they may have learned about from their parents or grandparents. If feasible, involve the parents or grandparents in such events. Help the children sharpen their awareness of the link between the generations and encourage communication and warm feelings between children and older people. Religious or ethnic holidays are a good way to teach the history or the meaning of these traditions with ceremonial foods. Nature's rhythm of life and death open up all sorts of opportunities for wonderful projects.

What can you do in the winter?

Look for animal tracks on the snow.

Remember to feed the birds.

Use "leather breeches" (dried string beans) in a hot soup or stew.

Have a memory day of the things you did last summer. Bring in souvenirs and tell about them.

Have the children decide how the class could be represented in a past and present poster. Use symbols that represent special people and events such as old records, clothing, knick-knacks, books, photographs, etc. Make collages and class murals of all the things you want to remember about the past year using postcards, pictures, fabrics. Add hand and feet prints, weight and height charts, favorite colors, pictures or labels of favorite foods, items collected on vacations and hikes. When the masterpiece is completed, post on the wall. Prepare and serve a good food that was discovered in the past year; add the recipe to your collage. Do this each year for a class history record. Family records could be designed this way also.

January 6th-Twelfth Night Party

Invite friends to celebrate with you. Ask them to bring something to share. A gift that reveals something about the person such as a favorite poem, a song, food, a game, a story. Use colored paper, scissors and string to make beautiful designs to resemble the heavens, stars, moon, planets and snowflakes for decorations. Make a:

Sesame Cake

2 cups whole wheat flour
1 cup enriched white flour
1/2 teaspoon salt
2 teaspoons baking powder
1/2 cup toasted sesame seeds
1/2 cup brown sugar

1/4 cup soft margarine
2 eggs
1 teaspoon grated lemon rind
1 1/2 cups milk
1 teaspoon untoasted sesame seeds
3 whole almonds or beans

Sift flour, salt and baking powder together and mix with the toasted sesame seeds and almonds or beans. Cream margarine and sugar together until fluffy. Blend in lemon rind and milk. Add the flour mixture all at once, mixing until blended. Do not overmix. Turn the mixture into a well greased, lightly floured 9" round pan. Sprinkle the untoasted sesame seeds over the top. Bake for 70 minutes at 350°F. Cool. Cover with a thin layer of your favorite frosting. Decorate like a crown using bits of red and green apple, orange and lemon rind, nuts and seeds.

Recite a blessing and serve the cake with mulled cider. The three people who find the almonds or beans are hailed as the "Wise Men" and immediately don the most exquisite robes available (colorful old drapes, capes or ponchos make great robes). Use construction paper cut in the form of a crown. Use colored shapes of glazed paper for jewels. After the coronation, the royal persons rule the party. Their subjects share their gifts.

January 7th

In 1896, the first Fanny Farmer Cook Book was published. Try the Cottage Cheese Pancakes for breakfast in the present edition. Pour the batter into a pitcher; pour out all sorts of beautiful designs on the griddle (stars, flowers, cats). Pour the batter through a funnel and make great shapes. Delicious with apricots!

January 15th—Martin Luther King's Birthday

In December of 1955, a black woman named Rosa Parks refused to give her seat on a city bus to a white person. That started a new battle in the long struggle for the rights of blacks in the United States. For the next 12 years, their leader was Martin Luther King, Jr. Try some "Soul Foods" in his memory, such as:

Sweet Potato Pie

Pastry for 9" nut pie crust
(See Miscellaneous Recipes)
2 pounds yams
1/2 cup soft margarine
1 teaspoon cinnamon
1/2 teaspoon ginger

1/8 teaspoon salt
1/2 cup brown sugar
3 eggs, separated
1/4 cup lemon juice
1/2 cup lowfat milk
1/2 cup orange juice

Boil the yams until just done, peel, and mash thoroughly. Add the margarine, spices, salt and sugar to the hot yams. Beat until light and smooth. Beat the egg yolks until light and add to the yam mixture. Stir in the lemon juice, orange juice and milk, mixing well. Beat the egg whites until very stiff and fold them into the filling gently. Pour into the uncooked pastry shell and bake at 450°F for 10 minutes. Reduce the heat to 350°F and bake 25 to 35 minutes longer, or until the pie is puffed up and firm in the middle.

Chinese New Year

Have an oriental party. Sprout and serve bean sprouts in a salad or sandwiches. Have a discussion around a fire on what you know about China and its contribution to civilization.

Egg Foo Yung

1 medium green pepper, chopped
1 medium onion, chopped
1 cup cooked, deveined shrimp,
chopped

1 cup bean sprouts, drained
2-3 tablespoons soy sauce
5 eggs
1 can (5 ounces) sliced water chestnuts, well drained

Heat just enough oil to cover the bottom of a heavy skillet. Saute the green pepper and onion until tender. Stir in shrimp, water chestnuts, bean sprouts and soy sauce. Heat mixture. Remove from heat. Beat eggs until thick, about 5 minutes. Blend shrimp-vegetable mixture into eggs. Heat additional oil to cover the bottom of the skillet. Pour mixture from a soup ladle or cup into skillet forming patties. When brown on one side, turn over. Patties may be kept warm until serving time between folds of a towel in warm oven. Serve with "Hot Soy Sauce (see below). Makes about sixteen 2 1/2 inch patties.

Hot Soy Sauce

Make paste of 2 tablespoons cornstarch and 1/4 cup cold water. Stir into 2 cups boiling soup stock, bouillon or consomme, and 2 tablespoons soy sauce. Cook, stirring constantly until clear and thickened.

February 14th—St. Valentine's Day

Try exchanging "life cake" valentines instead of valentine cards with your friends. In centuries past, gingerbread "life cakes" were molded in old prized decorated molds. You can use heart-shaped cookie cutters or cut a heart-shape out of cardboard and use a toothpick to trace around the cardboard placed on the dough. Decorate the unbaked cookies with almonds and raisins. Write messages, too.

Valentine Gingerbread

1 cup soft margarine	1/4 teaspoon cloves
1/2 cup sugar	1/2 teaspoon salt
4 cups whole wheat flour	1/4 teaspoon mace
1 teaspoon ginger	3/4 cup dark molasses

Cream sugar and margarine. Add sifted dry ingredients alternately with molasses. Roll on floured board. Cut into shapes. Bake at 300° F. for 30 minutes.

February 22nd—George Washington's Birthday

Try a cherry parfait. Repeat layers of vanilla custard and cherries in parfait or sherbet glasses. Make oatmeal cookies in the shape of hatchets and add to the top of each parfait.

In 1630, Indians introduced *popcorn* to the Pilgrims. Make popcorn and invite your friends to share it.

What can you do in the spring?

Look for signs of new life, new color, new birds and butterflies. Celebrate National Nutrition Week or Food Day by trying wholesome new foods.

Purim Day

According to legend, Haman, the villain of the Purim story, who tried to annihilate all Jews in Persia, wore a three-cornered hat. Celebrate Purim by eating *Hamantaschen,* the little three-sided pastries filled with all sorts of good things. You will find the Purim story in the Book of Esther.

Hamantaschen

The Pastry
2 cups flour, enriched
2 teaspoons baking powder
1/2 cup sugar
1/2 teaspoon salt
2 eggs, well beaten
3 tablespoons corn oil
1 lemon rind, grated (optional)

The Filling
2 cups ground poppy seed
1/3 cup honey
1 egg
1 tablespoon lemon juice
4 tablespoons chopped nuts or
As a filling, use cooked and
    mashed prunes or apricots.

Sift the dry ingredients together. Add the eggs, oil and rind. Mix well. Roll out dough to 1/4" thickness. Cut into 3" squares. Wash poppy seeds in hot water. Mix with honey and cook over low heat for five minutes. Remove from heat and add other ingredients. Place filling on each square and fold into triangles. Press edges together. Bake at 375°F for 20 minutes.

March 17th—St. Patrick's Day

Delight your family or class with an Irish party. Put on your touch of green and decorate with shamrocks using green paper napkins. Read Irish poetry, sing Irish songs and dance Irish jigs. Serve:

Irish Soda Bread

2 cups whole wheat flour
1 cup enriched flour
1 1/2 teaspoon salt
3/4 teaspoon soda
1/2 cup corn oil
1/4 cup brown sugar

1/4 cup molasses
1 egg
1 1/2 cups sour milk or buttermilk
1 1/2 cups currants
1 1/2 cups raisins

Preheat oven to 325°F. Sift or mix together dry ingredients. Cream oil, sugar and molasses together. Beat in egg. Add alternately dry ingredients with sour milk. Stir in fruit. Pour batter into greased 8 x 4 x 2 1/2" loaf pan. Bake about 75 minutes.

Mardi Gras

Mardi Gras is French for Fat Tuesday. It is the day for a wild celebration before Lent begins. On one of the days just before Lent begins, plan a party with games. Lent is a big contest between winter and spring, so get ready with your own contests. Have sack races, three-legged races, wheelbarrow races, balloon races and tests of strength.

Passover Time

The Jewish holiday of Passover is a celebration of liberation, the exodus from Egypt. It is as meaningful today as it has been throughout history—a celebration of freedom. Ceremonial foods include:

Three Matzos—symbolize the haste of the departure of the Jewish people

197

from Egypt. There was no time to leaven the bread. Three matzos also represent the ancient Jewish religious groupings.

Roasted Shankbone—Symbol of the pascal lamb offered in sacrifice at the Temple.

Roasted Egg—The second offering brought to the Temple on Passover. The egg also symbolizes the cycle of life and death, freedom and oppression.

Bitter Herbs (Horseradish)—The symbol of the bitterness of slavery.

Charoses—Made from apples, raisins and sweet wine to resemble the mortar used in laying the bricks for the pyramids. It also symbolizes the sweetness of freedom.

Karpas—A green vegetable (parsley). The green is a reminder that Passover coincides with the arrival of spring and new life. In ancient times, Passover was an agricultural festival; an occasion for giving thanks.

See Chapter XII of Exodus in the Bible.

Charoses

*6 medium apples, grated or
    chopped very fine*
1/2 cup raisins (optional)

1/2 teaspoon cinnamon
1/4 cup sweet wine
1/2 cup chopped nuts

Mix and serve.

Easter

The Easter season is the time for the celebration of new life—springtime. Decorate eggs. Pick fresh flowers. Try the traditional Russian Easter bread:

Koulitchey—Resurrection Bread

2 cups milk
8-10 cups whole wheat flour
*2 packages yeast (dissolved in
    1/3 cup warm water)*
1/4 cup corn oil

1/2 cup brown sugar
1 teaspoon salt
2 eggs
*2 cups raisins, nuts, currants (op-
    tional)*

Prepare dough in conventional or sponge method. Oil coffee cans for molds. Fill about two-thirds full with dough. Let rise. Bake in oven at 375°F for about 60 minutes. When cool, frost with cream cheese mixed with lemon juice. Decorate with orange, lime or lemon rind. Use a vegetable peeler for long strips. Shape into flower petals. Use nuts for flower centers. Serve for Easter breakfast.

April 6th

Robert Perry reached the North Pole on this day. Commemorate the great sense of adventure and perserverance with a family or class hike along new trails. Pack a picnic lunch.

April is a time for planting

Watch new life spring from the earth. Phone your local Agricultural Extension Service for information on gardens, soils and composting. Plant a mini-garden of wheat, lettuce, spinach, tomatoes, string beans and radishes. Radishes are ready to eat in about two weeks after planting. If you don't have a yard, try herbs in pots on the window sill or window boxes or bushel baskets on a balcony or patio. Easy to grow and delicious herbs are parsley, basil, savory, dill and chives.

Wild foods are abundant in April

Have an "Edible Wild Food Day". Edible wild foods are fun to gather and eat for a new tasting experience. Some plants are poisonous, so be sure to consult a local expert. Perhaps you could organize an expedition with a park naturalist or your biology teacher. Dandelion greens make an interesting addition to salads. The top shoots of young ferns are delicious as cooked greens. Young shoots of poke weed are called "wild asparagus" and are a delicacy (take care not to eat older parts of the plant).

May—Senior Citizens' Month

Invite a senior citizen to your class or home for dinner. Find out his or her favorite foods from the olden days. Prepare an old-fashioned favorite and one of your new specialties.

Mother's Day

Have the class plan a special treat to take home to Mother. Perhaps you would like to use one of the recipes in the Miscellaneous Section, or have the children bring one of their mother's favorite recipes from home and let the class choose which one they'd like to try. Poems or songs could also be made on homemade cards for a special surprise.

May 25th—Africa Freedom Day

This day marks the organization of an annual celebration of African unity. The daily bread and potatoes of Africa are cassova, rice and corn. Yams, plantains, rice and millet are basic to the diet in some parts of Africa. Try this super-nutritious recipe from Ghana called:

African Liver and Yams

1 pound liver	*1 teaspoon salt*
2 medium yams or sweet potatoes	*1 teaspoon oil*
1 medium onion	*1 medium tomato*
1 cup water	

Cut liver into small cubes. Soak in hot water for 10 minutes. Peel and cut yams and onion in cubes. Cook in a small amount of water until tender. Add the liver, chopped tomato, salt, pepper and oil to yams. Simmer for 10 minutes. Serve.

Memorial Day

Have the children pick fresh flowers or make some at school out of colored paper. Egg cartons can also be used by cutting out the sections. See Arts and Crafts Activity Section. Plan a picnic with sandwiches and other food in a basket lined with the flowers. Discuss the meaning of Memorial Day on the picnic.

What can you do in the summer?

Visit gardens, pick string beans and dry them.

Have an ice cream social at school.

Set up an orange juice stand. Sell the juice to visitors.

Pack a picnic basket and hike along a trail.

Find a fish pond and go fishing.

Father's Day

Let Dad sleep late this morning (Mom, too!) The children can get up early and quietly start to fix a delicious breakfast. Maybe waffles or pancakes topped with fruit would be good. When everything is ready, ring a bell throughout the house, calling everybody to the celebration.

July 4th—Independence Day

A traditional way of preparing eggs for a Fourth of July picnic is done by serving:

Pink Eggs

Shell hard-cooked eggs. Place them in a bowl with juice drained from a jar of pickled beets. Chill eggs, turning occasionally until pink on all sides. Remove eggs from beet juice and dry with paper toweling. Serve eggs chilled with salt and pepper. For a tart relish, serve the pickled beets.

You also might try preparing a *Star Cake*. Bake one of the cakes found in the Miscellaneous Section in layer pans and let cool. On one layer, space 5 toothpicks, 4 1/2" apart around the outside edge to mark the star points. About 2 1/2" in from the edge, place 5 more toothpicks, spacing them evenly between every two of the outside toothpicks. Cut out pieces of cake, cutting from the outside to the inside toothpicks in order to form star points. Frost the star and cut out pieces. Place the star in the center of a serving plate and arrange the cake pieces with the rounded sides toward the center, around the star.

Plan a list for a *scavenger hunt* and include common and unusual foods to find on the hunt. The group who returns first with all the items on the list is the winner!

Pick *berries* and eat them in salads, fruit cups and as toppings on your ice cream for a very special treat.

Make a *fruit basket*. Have a Fondue Party with a fresh fruit basket. Make the basket by going up and down with a knife in a zig-zag fashion around the circumference of a watermelon, cantaloupe or honeydew melon. Clean out the seeds. Use the leftover fruit for melon balls or cubes. Fill the fruit basket with chunks of a variety of fruit—grapes, apples, peaches, oranges, etc. Decorate with mint. Enjoy this treat as an appetizer or dessert. Have family and friends sit around the table to spear the fruit with fondue forks or toothpicks. Delectable!

What can you do in the fall?

Visit apple, peach and plum orchards and pick fruit.

Corn fields and pumpkin patches are inviting.

Gather leaves such as mint and herbs; dry them for flavoring tea.

Fourth Friday in September—American Indian Day

About this time of the year, the Indians would gather seeds for the next year's crops. Why not take a family or class hike and see what kinds of seeds you can find. Can you identify the tree, the shrub or the plant, the fruit from the plant or the leaf? Perhaps you would like to pick some herbs like wild mint and hang it up to dry. Use it for tea or flavoring during the winter. Try corn pudding, Indian pudding or a corn roast in the back yard.

Corn Pudding

2 cups drained whole kernel corn
  (canned or cooked frozen or fresh)
1 teaspoon sugar
1/2 teaspoon salt
1/4 teaspoon pepper

2 eggs, well beaten
1 cup lowfat milk
1 tablespoon soft margarine
2 tablespoons cracker crumbs

Heat oven to 350°F. Mix ingredients thoroughly. Pour into greased 1 quart baking dish. Set in pan of hot water 1" deep. Bake 60 to 70 minutes or until a knife inserted 1" from the edge comes out clean. Serves 8.

Indian Pudding

4 cups lowfat milk
2/3 cups molasses
2/3 cup yellow corn meal
1/3 cup brown sugar

1/2 teaspoon salt
3/4 teaspoon cinnamon
3/4 teaspoon nutmeg
1/4 cup soft margarine

Heat oven to 300°F. Heat 3 cups of milk and molasses in saucepan. Combine corn meal, sugar, salt and spices. Gradually stir into hot liquid. Add margarine. Cook over low heat stirring frequently until mixture thickens, about 10 minutes. Pour into greased 2 quart baking dish. Pour remaining cup of cold milk over pudding. Do not stir. Bake for 3 hours. Serves 8.

Second Week of October—School Lunch Week

Pass your ideas for better lunches on to your school board. Make Munchies for the lunch bags and for snacks using sunflower seeds, nuts and raisins.

October 12th—Columbus Day

Celebrate with an easy Italian treat by serving:

Pizza

English Muffins
Tomato sauce

Parmesan cheese
Cheddar or part-skim Mozzarella
  cheese

Top each muffin half with about 2 teaspoons of tomato sauce and 2 tablespoons of grated cheese. Sprinkle with Parmesan cheese. Bake in oven for 15 to 20 minutes at 350°F.

October 31st—Halloween

Make a *jack-o-lantern* to look like your favorite person.

Pumpkin Seeds

Place the pulp from the pumpkin in a colander and rinse the pulp from the seeds. Put the seeds on a cookie sheet, sprinkle with corn oil and roast at 350°F for 30 minutes.

Cheese Pumpkins

Soften cheddar cheese, moisten with salad dressing and shape into tiny balls. Roll in paprika, score with a toothpick at 1/4" intervals and flatten at top and bottom. Stick a raisin in the top for a pumpkin stem.

November—Birthday Anyone?

For your next birthday party, make portraits on sandwiches of all your guests. Play a "Who Am I" game. Cut sliced whole wheat bread with a glass, cookie cutter or knife into round, square, oval or pear shapes. Spread with peanut butter or cheese. Use carrot curls, parsley or coconut for hair. Nuts, raisins, apple pieces, banana chunks, etc. can be used for the eyes, nose and mouth. Guess whose portraits are on the sandwiches. Use leftover bread for puddings, stuffing or dry crumbs.

Fourth Thursday of November—Thanksgiving Day

Thanksgiving is a time to be grateful for all our blessings. This time evolved from the Pilgrims who planted their gardens with seeds to grow their own food. Although they experienced difficult times, they were thankful for the crops they raised. Celebrate this day by trying the Homemade Pumpkin Pie or Pudding recipe in the Miscellaneous Section.

Chanukah—Festival of Lights

The Jewish holiday of Chanukah is a celebration of religious freedom and is celebrated for eight days. Each evening as the blessing is said, another candle is added to the one lit the evening before until eight candles burn in the Menorah. The ninth candle is called a "shamash" and is used to light the others. This is a good time to discover some traditional Jewish dishes such as blintzes or latkes.

Potato Latkes (Pancakes)

2 cups grated raw potatoes
   (measure after draining)
2 eggs, beaten
1/2 teaspoon salt

2 tablespoons flour or matzo meal
1/4 teaspoon baking powder
1 small onion, grated (optional)

Combine and mix ingredients well. Drop by tablespoonful onto hot, greased skillet. Flatten to taste. Fry on both sides until brown. Serve with sour cream or applesauce.

Note: In order to save time or when working with younger children, prepare most of the grated potatoes ahead of time. Keep the potatoes covered with water until ready to use. Then drain. Have the children grate one or two potatoes and an onion for the experience of grating.

December—A Time for Sharing

Many parents do not have enough money to feed their families. Some have only half or less of what they need for a good, healthy diet. Older people and families with only one parent often have the least. Find out from the Welfare Department how much a family on welfare has to live on. Perhaps you could take time to write to your governor and let him know how you feel about families who go hungry. The governor can see to it that poor people have enough to live on. What can you share with a needy family?

Visit friends and neighbors and bring them something you've made at home or school for holiday celebrations. Share candles, pomander balls, baskets of goodies (nuts, fruits, cheeses), holiday bread, a picture or wall hanging. Bring your homemade musical instruments, bells, etc., to sing songs of good cheer as you approach the door of houses you are visiting. You may find this to be one of the most exciting experiences of the year.

December 25th—Christmas Day

Christmas is the time of year to show peace and goodwill toward fellow men. Try foods from different countries, especially breads which are a universal food. Eggnog is a traditional drink at this time of the year. (See Beverages in Recipe Section.)

Jule Kage—Christmas Bread from Norway

1/4 cup warm water	1/2 teaspoon cardamon
1 package active dry yeast	1 egg
3/4 cup lukewarm lowfat milk	2 tablespoons soft margarine
(scalded then cooled)	1/2 cup seedless raisins
1/2 cup sugar	1/3 cup citron, cut-up (optional)
1/2 teaspoon salt	3 1/4 to 3 1/2 cups flour, enriched

In bowl, dissolve yeast in water. Stir in rest of ingredients except half of flour. Mix until smooth. Add rest of flour until easy to handle. Turn onto lightly floured board; knead until smooth. Round up in greased bowl; cover and let rise until double, about 1 1/2 hours. Punch down; let rise again about 45 minutes. Shape into round loaf; place in greased 9" pie pan or on greased baking sheet. Cover, let rise 45 minutes. Brush with Egg Yolk Glaze: Mix with fork 1 egg yolk and 2 tablespoons cold water. Bake loaf at 350°F. for 30 to 40 minutes.

Christmas Tree Bread

Make Jule Kage recipe. After dough rises, divide dough in two (one for each tree). Form each into 17 1 1/2" balls. Arrange on slightly greased baking sheet in a 5, 4, 3, 2, 1 pattern and with 2 balls rolled together for the trunk. Let rise until double, 20 to 30 minutes. Heat oven to 350°F. and bake for 20 to 30 minutes, or until golden brown. Decorate with cream cheese icing, dried fruits and nuts. Makes 2 large trees.

Teacher's Note:

The celebrations presented in this section are cultural celebrations not intended as religious expression. Cultural celebrations are a great way to understand, appreciate and enjoy our own traditions as well as others.

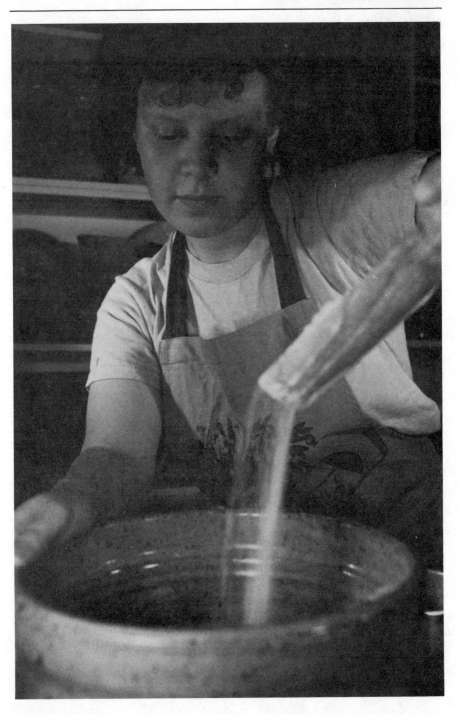

Introduction

The recipes in this section will help you create a dazzling variety of tasty, exotic, and nutritious dishes. The emphasis on nutrition is a departure from most recipes intended to delight children. All too often children are encouraged to eat sweet, salty, and greasy foods. Medical researchers have shown, to the dismay of many of us, that many traditional foods promote numerous serious health problems.

In December, 1977, the U.S. Senate Select Committee on Nutrition and Human Needs published the Second Edition of Dietary Goals for the United States. This report noted that in the past 50 years our diets have changed radically. The proportion of fatty, cholesterol, rich, salty and highly processed foods in our diets has risen markedly. These changes have had a profound effect on our health. Six out of ten of the major causes of death and disability in the U.S. have been directly linked to the food we eat. The diet-related illnesses include heart disease, artery disease, cancer, high blood pressure, diabetes and cirrhosis of the liver. Obesity, tooth decay, periodontal disease are additional conditions significantly influenced by diet. Death and disability from diet-related diseases account for about half of all deaths. These diseases and conditions are multifactorial in their etiologies; nevertheless, diet is one important factor that is easily modified because it is under personal control. Eating well is one way to demonstrate power to choose and obtain good food, as well as respect for one's body.

To children the quality and kind of food offered is one way of expressing awareness, concern and love. Highly advertised "junk foods" or peer pressure should not determine food fare for children. Those responsible for the care of children need to be conscious of their present and future health. Children are building their bodies for life; genes set the architectural plans, the building materials are the food they eat. The quality of food eaten has a direct relationship to the quality of health. Ethnicity, personal preferences, and individual needs should be considered and respected as an expression of one's uniqueness.

Parents and teachers should be accurately informed of the relationship between early eating habits and the development of diet-related diseases later in life. Eating habits which condition children to consume highly processed foods, or foods high in fat, sugar, and salt are not only physiologically unhealthy, but are also developmentally detrimental by instilling in children a taste for foods that do not support good health.

Those involved with nurturing the body, mind and spirit of children will find the U.S. Dietary Goals a useful and timely baseline for feeding their families and planning food programs.

In July, 1979, the Surgeon General of the United States—our nation's top health official—issued a report entitled *Healthy People*. This report, like the earlier Senate report, urged that Americans eat a diet lower in cholesterol, saturated fat, sugar, and salt.

Most of the recipes in this section are in line with the U.S. Dietary Goals and the Surgeon General's advice. The modest number of recipes that are rich in fat, cholesterol, sugar, or salt should be used sparingly.

U.S. Dietary Goals

1. To avoid overweight, consume only as much energy (calories) as is expended; if overweight, decrease energy intake and increase energy expenditure.

2. Increase the consumption of complex carbohydrates and "naturally occuring" sugars from about 28 percent of energy intake to about 48 percent of energy intake.

3. Reduce the consumption of refined and processed sugars by about 45 percent to account for about 10 percent of total energy intake.

4. Reduce overall fat consumption from approximately 40 percent to about 30 percent of energy intake.

5. Reduce saturated fat consumption to account for about 10 percent of total energy intake; and balance that with poly-unsaturated and mono-unsaturated fats, which should account for about 10 percent of energy intake each.

6. Reduce cholesterol consumption to about 300 mg. a day.

7. Limit the intake of sodium by reducing the intake of salt to about 5 grams a day.

The Goals Suggest the Following Changes in Food Selection and Preparation:

1. Increase consumption of fruits and vegetables and whole grains.

2. Decrease consumption of refined and other processed sugars and foods high in such sugars.

3. Decrease consumption of foods high in total fat, and partially replace saturated fats, whether obtained from animal or vegetable sources, with poly-unsaturated fats.

4. Decrease consumption of animal fat, and choose meats, poultry and fish which will reduce saturated fat intake.

5. Except for young children, substitute low-fat and non-fat milk for whole milk, and low-fat dairy products for high fat dairy products.

6. Decrease consumption of butterfat, eggs and other high cholesterol sources. Some consideration should be given to easing the cholesterol goal for pre-menopausal women, young children and the elderly in order to obtain the nutritional benefits of eggs in the diet.

7. Decrease consumption of salt and foods high in salt content.

Persons with physical and/or mental ailments who have reason to believe that they should not follow guidelines for the general population should consult with a health professional having expertise in nutrition, regarding their individual case.

Beverages

Ambrosia Shake

4 sliced ripe bananas
1/2 cup orange juice
1/4 teaspoon vanilla
4 cups reconstituted nonfat dry milk
(use 1 cup ice cubes for 1 cup water)

Blend in blender. 6 servings.

Honey Hug

2 cups skim or lowfat milk
2 teaspoons honey
1 teaspoon vanilla
Sprinkle of cinnamon

Heat milk, honey, and vanilla. Sprinkle with cinnamon before serving.

Silky Milky

1 quart buttermilk
3 cups orange juice
1/2 teaspoon cinnamon
1/3 cup lemon juice
1 tablespoon honey (optional)

Blend ingredients.

Sassy Lassy

4 cups cold water
1 1/4 cup nonfat dry milk
4 tablespoons molasses
1/2 teaspoon nutmeg

Mix together, shake well.

Frosty Fruit Froths

2 peeled oranges
2 peeled bananas
2 cups crushed ice or 1 full tray of
cubes
2 cups apple juice
1/2 teaspoon cinnamon

Blend in blender (gradually add ice cubes). Sprinkle cinnamon on top.

Og Nog

1 well beaten egg
1 teaspoon sugar
1 cup skim or lowfat milk
1/4 teaspoon vanilla

Beat egg and sugar together. Beat in milk and vanilla. Sprinkle with nutmeg.

Buttermilk

3/4 cup nonfat dry milk
3 3/4 cups warm water
1/2 cup buttermilk (may be homemade)

Sprinkle nonfat dry milk over warm water and stir. Add buttermilk, cover and let stand at room temperature 8 hours. Stir until smooth, cover and refrigerate. Makes about 1 quart.

Nutty Juices

1/2 cup nonfat dry milk
1 cup orange juice
1 1/2 cup pineapple juice
1/2 cup blanched almonds
1 cup ice

Blend in blender. (Add ice gradually.) Sprinkle with nutmeg.

Snippy Sippy

4 cups tomato juice
4 long stems of green onions

Trim and wash stems. Sip juice through stem.

Slumber Under

2 cups lowfat milk
1 cup cider
3 sticks cinnamon

Heat milk and cider. Stir with a cinnamon stick.

Strawberry Swallow

1 1/2 cup dry nonfat milk
2 cups fresh or frozen berries
1 teaspoon vanilla
1 cup water
1 tray of ice cubes

Blend in blender. (Add ice gradually).

Spice Apple Sipper

1 cup yogurt
3/4 cup ice cubes
1 cup stewed apples
1/2 teaspoon cinnamon

Blend in blender. Sprinkle with nutmeg.

Peanut Smoothie

2 cups nonfat milk
4 ice cubes
1/2 teaspoon cinnamon
1/3 cup peanut butter
1 tablespoon molasses

Blend in blender. Or omit ice and serve heated.

Hot Mulled Cider

1 quart cider
3 whole cloves
2 whole allspice
2 sticks cinnamon
1/2 teaspoon ground nutmeg

Combine and simmer for 30 minutes. (Put allspice and cloves in tea ball.)

Golden Cow

1 can frozen orange juice (6 oz.)
1 cup nonfat dry milk
1 teaspoon vanilla
1 cup water
2 1/2 cups ice cubes

Blend in blender (add ice cubes gradually).

Strawberry Frappe Forever

1 cup lowfat or skim milk
1/4 cup fresh or frozen berries
1 scoop vanilla or strawberry ice cream

Blend milk and berries. Before serving, add ice cream.

Festive Frosty Flurries

1. Combine 2 cups lowfat yogurt with 4 cups of pineapple juice. Blend 1/2 cup shredded coconut. Top with a slice of orange.
2. Blend 2 bananas with 1/2 cup grape juice, 3 cups lowfat milk, 1 cup ice cubes. Sprinkle shredded coconut on top.
3. Combine equal amounts of apple juice and lowfat milk, sprinkle with cinnamon.

4. Blend one part orange juice, 2 parts cantaloupe, juice of one lemon, 2 cups crushed ice. Garnish with mint leaves.
5. Blend equal amounts of watermelon, ice cubes, dash of honey, dash of lemon juice, and garnish with mint leaves.
6. Combine equal amounts of grapefruit and cranberry juices. Stir and garnish with spoonful of lowfat yogurt and a sprig of mint (optional).
7. Blend 3 cups of pineapple juice, 2 cubed large carrots and 1 cup ice cubes.
8. Combine 2 cups buttermilk, 2 cups canned pineapple juice; chill. Garnish with a sprig of mint.
9. Blend 1 cup blackberries, 1 cup lowfat yogurt and 1 cup ice cubes.

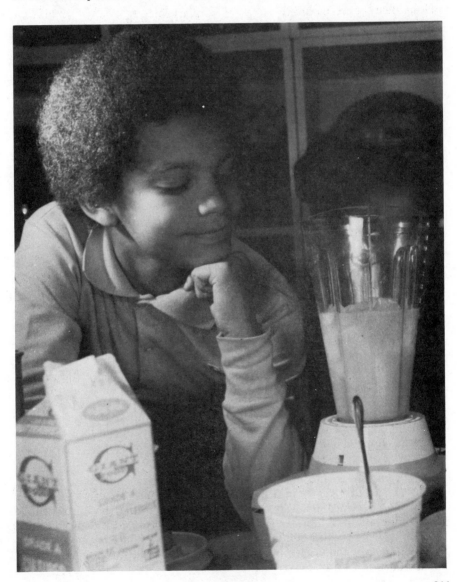

Salads

Cool Slaw

1 cup lowfat yogurt
2 tablespoons vinegar or lemon juice
1 carrot, grated
1/8 teaspoon salt

1/4 cup mayonnaise
3 cups cabbage

Wash cabbage; place in refrigerator until crisp; shred; grate carrot. Combine yogurt, mayonnaise, salt, and vinegar or lemon juice. Mix thoroughly with cabbage and carrot. Serves 6.

Creole Potato Salad

6 cold boiled potatoes
2 young green onions
1 large stalk celery
1/2 teaspoon black pepper
1/2 teaspoon salt

1/2 cup boiled salad dressing
(see page 219)
2 hard-boiled eggs
2 green peppers
1/2 lemon or lime, squeezed

Slice potatoes, cut celery fine, chop all other ingredients, mix with the salad dressing in bowl, add pepper, salt, juice 1/2 lemon or lime, and mix. Chill for two hours, then serve generous portions on large lettuce leaf. Serves 6.

Cumin Cucumber Salad

1 medium-sized cucumber, chopped
1 small onion, chopped fine (1/3 cup)
1 tomato, chopped into 16ths
a few sprigs of parsley, chopped

1 teaspoon cumin seeds
1/2 cup lowfat cottage cheese
1/2 cup lowfat yogurt

Chop the cucumber into half-inch sticks. Add the onion and tomato to the cucumber and toss gently in a bowl. Toast the cumin seeds in a small dry frying pan over medium heat only until they are brittle, not browned, It should take about 1 minute. Place the cottage cheese and yogurt in your blender, add the toasted cumin, and buzz until the mixture is smooth. Pour the dressing over the vegetables, toss gently, and refrigerate for an hour, if possible, before serving. Serves 4.

Cuke-A-Doodle Doo

2 cucumbers, sliced very thin
2 tablespoons lemon juice
1/8 teaspoon pepper
chives

1 cup lowfat yogurt
1 tablespoon finely chopped onion
parsley, chopped
salt to taste (optional)

Mix ingredients together. Chill 1 hour or more to blend the flavors. Serves 4.

Indian Adventure

2 cups pineapple chunks (canned in
its own juice) or 1 fresh pineapple
2 tomatoes, firm and large
1/2 teaspoon curry

2 1/2 cups cooked lentils (about 1
cup dried)
salt to taste
1 tablespoon oil

Heat oil in a skillet and add the spices to it. After a few minutes, add the cooked, drained lentils and mix them well with the heated spices. Cool. Cut the tomatoes into bite-size pieces. Mix together the chopped pineapple, the tomatoes, and the lentils. Serve with plain yogurt. Serves 6.

Lemon Bean Salad

2 cups dried white beans
1/4 cup lemon juice
1/2 teaspoon pepper
1/4 cup chopped chives

3-4 tablespoon oil
2 cloves garlic, minced
1 cup shredded lettuce

Cook beans (about 3 hours; 2 hours if soaked overnight). Mix together all the remaining ingredients, except the lettuce. Beat well and pour over the beans. Chill thoroughly. Serve on dark green lettuce or spinach. Serves 6.

Orange-Cauliflower Salad

4 oranges, sectioned
2 cups uncooked cauliflowerets
1/4 cup chopped green pepper
lettuce cups

2 cups bite-size pieces spinach
1/4 cup fruit or vegetable salad
dressing

Toss orange sections, cauliflowerets, green pepper, spinach and salad dressing. Makes 5 or 6 servings.

Peanut-Rice Salad

Combine:
3 cups brown rice, cooked and cooled
1/4 cup each red and green minced
sweet peppers

1/4 cup chopped green onions

Toss in dressing of:
3-4 tablespoons salad oil
3 tablespoons lemon juice

1/2 teaspoon sugar
1/2 teaspoon salt

Mount on spinach or dark green lettuce and surround with:
fresh orange sections   fresh pineapple slices

Sprinkle with 3/4 cup chopped roasted peanuts. Serves 6.

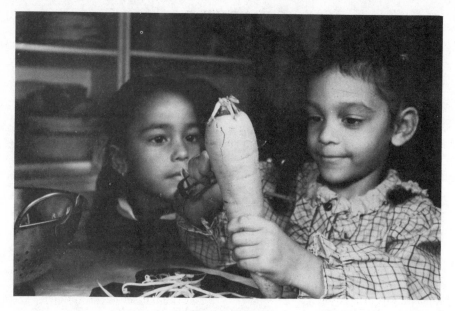

Rocket Salad

For each serving, place a crisp lettuce leaf on a salad plate.

Launching pad: 1 slice pineapple
Rocket: 1/2 peeled banana set upright in center of pineapple slice
Nose Cone: 1/2 cherry fastened to top of banana with toothpick

Spinach and Rice Salad

1/4 to 1/2 pound fresh spinach
1 small onion, thinly sliced
1/2 cup thinly sliced celery
1/4 cup sliced radishes
3 hard cooked eggs, sliced

1 1/2 cups cold, cooked brown rice
1/2 teaspoon salt
1/4 teaspoon pepper
French dressing

Wash spinach thoroughly. Break off stems and measure 1 quart. If leaves are large, tear into bite-sized pieces. Shake spinach in a towel to dry well. Arrange attractively with other vegetables, eggs, and rice in a salad bowl. Chill. When ready to serve, season, add dressing and toss lightly. Serves 5-6.

Spring Salad

3 cups lowfat cottage cheese
1/4 cup toasted sunflower seeds
1/4 cup toasted sesame seeds
1 carrot
1 medium tomato
1 large green pepper
1 cucumber

1 cup fresh alfalfa sprouts
1/4 teaspoon pepper
juice of 1/2 lemon
2 chopped, hard-cooked eggs
1 scallion
1 stalk celery
1/2 cup fresh parsley

Combine cottage cheese and seeds. Chill. Chop carrot, tomato, scallion, pepper, celery, cucumber and parsley into very small pieces. Combine. Mix with cheese mixture. Add remaining ingredients. Mix and Serve. Serves 6.

214

Sprouts Salad

1 cup alfalfa sprouts, loosely packed
1/2 cup sunflower seeds (optional)
2 or more cups salad greens, torn
  into bite size pieces
6 or 8 radishes, sliced

2-3 tablespoons sesame or olive oil
1-2 tablespoons cider vinegar
1/8 teaspoon salt
1/2 cucumber, sliced (peeled if
  waxed)

Toast sunflower seeds by stirring in a dry pan on medium heat for about 3 minutes; then toss together with greens, sprouts, radish, and cucumber. Mix oil, vinegar and salt to make dressing; add to salad and toss again. Serves 4-6.

Tabouli-Lebanese Salad

1/4 cup cooked dry navy or
  garbanzo beans (optional)
1 1/2 cups bulgur (cracked wheat), raw
3 cups boiling water
1 1/2 cup minced parsley
3/4 cup minced scallions
2 teaspoons dried mint

1 cucumber
2 medium tomatoes, chopped
1/2 cup lemon and/or lime juice
1/4 cup oil
1/2 teaspoon salt
Pepper to taste
Raw cabbage, lettuce or spinach
  leaves

Soak the bulgur in water for 15 minutes, until the wheat is light and fluffy. Drain excess water and shake in a strainer or press with hands to remove as much water as possible. Mix the bulgur, cooked beans, and remaining ingredients. Chill for at least one hour. Serve on raw leaves with garnish of fresh mint, alfalfa sprouts, green pepper, cucumber or tomato. Serves 6.

Three Bean Salad

1 1/2 cup cooked green string beans,
  cut into 1'' pieces
1 1/2 cup cooked yellow wax beans,
  cut into 1 '' pieces
1 1/2 cup cooked red kidney beans
1 1/2 cup cooked garbanzo beans or
  chick peas

1 large onion, sliced thin
1/3 cup oil
2/3 cup wine or cider vinegar
Salt and pepper to taste
2 teaspoons sugar (optional)
Chopped green pepper
Tarragon or basil to taste

Combine all the beans in a large mixing bowl. Mix the rest of the ingredients to make the dressing and pour it over the beans. Toss until everything is thoroughly combined. Cover the bowl and refrigerate overnight. Serves 6-8.

Three C's in Salad

1 cup cooked corn kernels, cut from
  the cob
1 tablespoon chopped green pepper
salt to taste (optional)
1/2 teaspoon dill

1 1/2 cups lowfat cottage cheese,
  well drained
1 tablespoon chopped parsley
1 stalk celery

Toss all ingredients together and store in a covered container in the refrigerator until serving time. Serves 4.

Tuna Crunch

1/2 cup lowfat yogurt
1/4 cup vinegar
2 tablespoons ketchup
1 small can tuna or salmon,
    preferably packed in water
1/2 cup cucumbers, chopped

1/2 cup bean sprouts
2 tablespoons green onions, chopped
Lemon juice to taste
1/2 cup celery, chopped
1 cup raw spinach, chopped
Tomato wedges

Beat yogurt, vinegar, ketchup, and lemon juice together. Drain and flake fish (or break up into bite-sized pieces), add vegetables. Stir in dressing.

Vegetable Falls

1 cup lowfat yogurt
3-4 cups mixed vegetables such as
    raw spinach, cucumber, cooked
    potatoes or eggplant
1/2 cup chopped onions

1 dried, crushed red chili pepper
2 tablespoons minced, fresh mint
    leaves
1/2 teaspoon salt (optional)
1/4 teaspoon black pepper

Combine ingredients and mix.

Waldorf Salad

4 apples, diced
1 cup walnut meats, chopped
1/2 cup raisins (optional)
a pinch of salt (optional)

4 stalks celery, cut in small pieces
1 cup lowfat yogurt (or boiled
    dressing see page 219)

Mix apples, celery, and nuts together with dressing. Serve on dark green lettuce leaves.

The Whole Plant Salad
Seeds, roots, stems, leaves and fruit

1 pound raw spinach
Salt (optional)
1 clove garlic, peeled
2 tablespoons lemon juice
4 tablespoons oil

Freshly ground black pepper
1 large ripe tomato, cut into wedges
1/2 red onion, sliced thin
1/2 cup toasted sesame seeds
1/2 cup sliced mushrooms

Wash the spinach well in several changes of clear water. Using a pair of scissors, cut away the tough stems and discard. Drain the spinach leaves and chill in a damp, clean cloth. Tear into bite-sized pieces. Rub the bottom of the bowl with the garlic. Add the lemon juice, oil, spinach, and sprinkle with pepper. Garnish with egg and tomato wedges and onion rings and toss lightly with a fork and spoon. Top with mushrooms and sesame seeds. Serves 6.

Winter Salad

3 cups lowfat cottage cheese
1/2 cup raisins
1/4 cup toasted sunflower seeds
1 tablespoon poppyseeds
1 tablespoon honey (optional)

2 chopped apples
1/4 cup chopped, toasted nuts, preferably almonds and/or cashews
Juice of 1/2 lemon

Combine everything. Serve very cold on greens. Garnish with bananas, apple wedges, or raisins. Serves 6.

Variations:
Fresh, firm pears; peaches; green, seedless grapes; orange sections; ripe honeydew; cantaloupe; pineapple.

Wedgies of Vegies

carrots
celery
broccoli flowerettes & shaved stems
zucchini or summer squash
cucumber
spinach or chard
scallions

red and green peppers
red cabbage
cauliflower
beets (peeled)
fresh green beans
radishes
tomatoes or raw mushrooms

Choose your favorites, chop into 1/2 inch wedges and top with alfalfa sprouts and dressing. Or cut into spears for dipping.

Fruit Salad Favorites*

Cut up orange sections or mandarin oranges and diced apple or banana slices, garnished with plain or toasted coconut.

Banana dipped in orange juice, rolled in toasted wheat germ (or coconut) and served with dollop of yogurt.

Banana slices, rolled in chopped peanuts, and pineapple spears.

Honeydew melon slices with balls of cantaloupe and watermelon.

Cut-up apples, oranges, bananas, grapes, and nuts blended with yogurt.

Pineapple slices or peach or pear halves topped with cottage cheese or yogurt.

Fresh or canned pineapple spears, strawberries and halves of blue plums.

Cantaloupe balls, Bing cherries, pineapple chunks.

Minted pineapple chunks, green grapes or halved Tokay grapes and cooked, diced celery root, garnished with toasted, slivered almonds.

Orange and grapefruit sections and avocado slices or slices of unpared red apples, garnished with pomegranate seeds or sliced strawberries.

Prunes or apricots stuffed with cottage cheese or peanut butter.

Sliced fresh pears and strawberries.

Pear or peach halves with nuts in hollow, topped with yogurt, ricotta or cottage cheese.

*Serve above salad combinations on salad greens with or without dressing.

Fresh peach slices, small green grapes and peanuts.

Diced fresh pineapple, strawberries and a sprinkling of finely chopped mint.

Vegetable Salad Variety*

Cooked green peas, cooked French-style green beans, chopped green pepper, onion and celery, marinated in oil-vinegar dressing overnight and garnished with pimiento.

Grated raw carrots and drained crushed pineapple or diced celery mixed with raisins.

Sliced zucchini, raw cauliflowerets or thinly sliced radishes with tossed greens.

Tomato sections, cucumber slices and cauliflowerets marinated in French dressing, each in its own little lettuce cup.

Cooked baby lima beans, sliced mushrooms and sliced green onions, seasoned with oregano.

Grated raw carrot, chopped sweet onion, chopped pepper, chopped celery, grated rind and sections of one orange and lettuce. Or grated raw parsnips, chopped sweet onion, celery and pimiento-stuffed olives tossed with greens.

Mound of cottage cheese with diced green or red pepper, cucumber and onions.

Asparagus tips on thick tomato slices, sprinkled with grated cheese.

Grated raw carrots and diced celery, mixed with raisins or nuts.

Halves of peeled, chilled tomatoes sprinkled with minced parsley, mint or chives. After dressing is added, sprinkle with grated sharp cheese.

Red cherry tomatoes, yellow plum tomatoes with unpared cucumber slices and sliced spring onions.

Overlapping slices of tomato, unpared cucumber slices and onion rings or slices.

Piquant Dressing

1/2 cup oil
1/4 cup red wine vinegar
2 tablespoons lemon juice
1/2 teaspoon dry mustard or 2
 teaspoons prepared mustard
Salt and black pepper

Optional:
2 tablespoons chopped parsley
2 tablespoons chopped onions or
 chives
2 teaspoons capers
1 clove garlic, crushed

Beat all ingredients together with rotary beater or shake well in tightly covered jar. Keep in a covered jar in refrigerator. Shake again before using as it separates on standing.

*Serve above salad combinations on salad greens with Piquant Dressing.

Dressings

Boiled Salad Dressing

1/2 teaspoon salt
1 tablespoon sugar
4 tablespoons flour
2 tablespoons butter
1/2 cup vinegar

2 teaspoons dry mustard
few grains cayenne pepper
2 eggs
1 1/2 cup lowfat milk

Sift and stir in the top part of a double boiler salt, mustard, sugar, pepper, flour. Slowly stir in eggs, milk, butter, and vinegar. Stir and cook over a double boiler until slightly thick. Cool. Serve on vegetable or fruit salad.

Dilled Yogurt Dressing

1 cup lowfat yogurt
2 tablespoons vinegar
1/2 small onion
1/4 teaspoon salt (optional)
1/2 teaspoon dill seeds

1/4 teaspoon dry mustard
1/4 teaspoon minced garlic or
  garlic powder
(pepper—optional)

Process all the ingredients in a blender until the onion is completely pureed.

Fruit Salad Dressing

1 cup lowfat yogurt
Ginger
Grated rind and juice 1/2 lemon

Nutmeg
Few pinches cinnamon
Honey (optional)

Mix together all the ingredients and add honey to taste. Chill.

Mayo (If You Must)

1 egg
1/2 teaspoon dry mustard
1/4 teaspoon salt

2 tablespoons vinegar or lemon juice
1 cup vegetable oil

For variety, add: basil, chives, dill, curry, parsley, caraway seeds, or finely chopped vegetables: scallions, green pepper, celery, mushrooms, sprouts.

Put everything but 3/4 cup of the oil in a blender and blend at medium speed. Add rest of oil slowly while blender is on. Keep refrigerated and use within 7 to 10 days.

Mock Thousand Island Dressing

1/2 cup lowfat yogurt
Lemon juice, a few drops

1/2 cup tomato juice (or less, depending on thickness desired)

Combine yogurt, tomato juice, and a little lemon juice. Blend or beat ingredients together. Vary by including chopped scallions, watercress, chives, dill, parsley. Minced garlic—let your taste determine the amount—will add a pleasant flavor to your dressings.

Soups

Brazilian Black Bean

2 cups dry black beans
3 1/2 cups water or stock
1 large, chopped onion
1 carrot, diced
lowfat yogurt
toasted sesame seeds

2 cups orange juice
2 cloves fresh garlic, crushed
1 stalk celery, diced
salt, black pepper
1/2 teaspoon ground cumin

Soak beans in water or stock for 4 hours. Cook beans 1 1/2 hours in covered pot. Add vegetables, garlic, orange juice, cumin, (you can increase or decrease amount) salt, and pepper. Simmer slowly at least 1 1/2 hours. Serve topped with yogurt and sesame seeds. Serves 6-8.

Cascadilla

4 cups tomato juice
1 cucumber, chopped
1 sweet pepper, chopped
1 scallion, chopped
1/2 teaspoon dill weed

1 cup lowfat yogurt
several fresh raw mushrooms
  thinly sliced
1 clove garlic, crushed
pepper

Combine and chill. Serve with croutons. Or garnish with watercress. Serves 4-6.

Cream of Tomato-Rice

7 fresh tomatoes quartered, or the
  equivalent canned
1 carrot, chopped
1 onion, chopped
1/2 cup celery, chopped
1 clove garlic, minced
2 tablespoons whole wheat flour

1/2-1 teaspoon salt
4 white peppercorns
1 teaspoon each oregano, basil
3/4 cup brown rice, cooked
3 cups vegetable stock or water
3 cups lowfat milk

Blend all ingredients but milk and rice in a blender. Add the rice. Simmer until flavors mingle. Add milk. Serves 6-8.

Cucumber Yogurt Soup

1 cup cold water
1/3 cup raisins
2 tablespoons scallions, chopped
salt and pepper

1/2 cup cucumber, chopped
3 cups lowfat yogurt
1/2 teaspoon fresh dill weed
1 tablespoon fresh parsley

Let raisins sit in cold water for 1/2 hour. Combine yogurt, scallions and cucumber. Add raisins and water. Garnish with parsley and dill. Serve very cold. Serves 4.

Fish Chowder

4 cups lowfat milk
1 tablespoon oil
1 medium onion
2 cups diced potatoes
1/2 cup diced carrots

1 cup water
1 pound fish (cod or haddock)
salt and pepper
garnish with chopped spinach

Heat oil in soup kettle. Add onion which had been thinly sliced, and cook until slightly browned. Add the cubed vegetables and water. Boil 5 minutes. Cut fish in small cubes, removing all the bones, and add to the mixture in the pot. Cook 15 minutes or until fish and vegetables are tender. Add the milk which has been scalded. Season to taste with salt and pepper, garnish with chopped spinach, and serve piping hot with crackers or croutons. Serves 6.

Fruit Sloop

3 cups fruit juice (unsweetened—
    orange, apple, pineapple, grape—
    your choice)
1/2 teaspoon dried mint
1 peach, peeled and chopped
honey (to taste)

1 banana, chopped
1 apple, peeled
juice from 1 lemon
pieces of fresh cantaloupe
1 cup lowfat yogurt or buttermilk

Combine all ingredients in blender. Thicken with more bananas or yogurt if you like it thick. Thin it with more fruit juice if you like it thin. Spice with dash of cinnamon, nutmeg or allspice. Top each serving with yogurt and a little fresh mint. Serves 8.

Gazpacho

5 cups tomato juice
3 fresh, diced tomatoes
1 small, diced cucumber (peeled)
juice of 1/2 lemon, 1/2 lime
1/2 teaspoon each tarragon, basil
dash of ground cumin
dash of tabasco sauce (or cayenne)
2 tablespoons oil (optional)

1 small onion, diced
1 chopped green pepper
2 scallions, chopped
2 tablespoons wine vinegar
    1/4 cup (packed) chopped, fresh
    fresh parsley
pepper to taste

Combine and chill. Serves 8.

Golden Squash Soup

1 small onion, sliced
1/4 cup flour
5 cups lowfat milk or 1 1/2 cup
   skim milk powder plus 5 cups water
1 1/2 cups cooked, pureed Hubbard
   squash

1/4 teaspoon celery salt
1/8 teaspoon curry powder
pepper as desired
2 tablespoons chopped parsley
oil for saute

Saute onion in a large saucepan for a few minutes. Blend flour with onion, add milk. Cook over low heat, stirring constantly until thickened. Remove from heat, gently blend in squash and seasoning. Heat to serving temperature, but do not boil. Sprinkle each serving of soup with parsley. Serves 6.

Lentil-Tomato Soupreme

2/3 cup dried lentils
4 cups water
1 onion, chopped
4 carrots, chopped
2 stalks celery, chopped
1 cup tomato paste

chopped parsley
garlic
salt and pepper
thyme
dill weed
tarragon

Put the first 5 ingredients into a large pot, salt and pepper and simmer gently for about 3 hours, replenishing the water as needed. Then add very small amounts of the herbs and spices according to taste. Stir in a cup of tomato paste and let it all heat through. Serves 6.

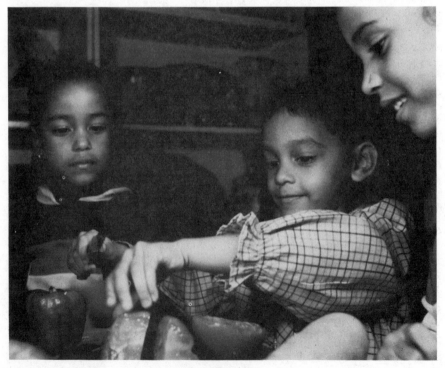

Mexican Bean Soup

1/2 cup navy beans
3 cups cold water
1 cup cooked corn
1 clove garlic, minced
1 onion, chopped
1 tablespoon parsley, chopped
oil for saute (optional)

1 cup celery, chopped
1/2 cup cabbage, finely shredded
2 teaspoons basil
1/8 teaspoon pepper
1 cup cooked tomatoes
salt to taste

Wash beans, place in large kettle and add water. Bring slowly to a boil and simmer until beans are tender. Saute the garlic, onion, parsley, celery, and cabbage in oil, and add to the bean mixture (or just add vegetables raw.) Stir thoroughly. Add spices, corn, and tomatoes and simmer about 30 minutes longer. Serves 6.

Minestrone

1 to 2 cups cooked chick peas
   (1/2 cup dry)
4 medium onions, chopped
3 cloves garlic, mashed
1 teaspoon oil (optional)
1 teaspoon oregano
1 quart home-canned or 6-8 fresh
   (chopped) tomatoes
1 handful raisins
1 small turnip, diced
2 cups green peas

3 cups cooked whole wheat noodles
   (1 cup uncooked)
1 teaspoon dried basil
a few pinches ground cinnamon
freshly ground black pepper
1 teaspoon salt
2 or 3 big carrots, diced
2 cups green snap beans
1/4 head cabbage
Dash red wine vinegar

Saute onions and garlic in a little oil or cook in a little water, adding spices and herbs except basil. Stir in tomatoes (with their juice). Cover the pot and begin to simmer the soup. Add water or stock if it starts getting thick. Add carrots and turnips and simmer 30 minutes (until firm). Add green beans and cook 20 minutes more. Now, add the chick peas with any extra water they were cooked in and cook until heated. Finally, add the peas, cabbage and noodles and cook a few more minutes. Add extra seasonings or vinegar to taste or extra water for desired thickness. Sprinkle with basil and parmesan, cheddar, ricotta or lowfat cottage cheese before serving. Serves 6-8.

Mushroom-Barley

6 1/2 cups vegetable stock or water
   with 1/2 teaspoon salt
3-4 tablespoons tamari (soy sauce)
2 cloves garlic, minced
1 1/2 pounds fresh mushrooms, sliced

1/2 cup raw pearled barley
1/4 cup lemon juice
1 medium onion, chopped
pepper

Cook barley in stock or water till tender. Add 5 cups additional stock or water, lemon juice, tamari, garlic, onion, mushrooms and fresh black pepper. Simmer 1 hour over very low heat. Sprinkle with freshly chopped scallions or chives just before serving. Serves 8.

Pea Bean Scene

3/4 cup dry navy (pea) beans
4 cups water
1 1/2 teaspoon salt
3/4 cup potatoes, diced
1/2 cup onion, chopped

1 1/2 teaspoon flour
1/2 tablespoon margarine
3/4 cup tomatoes, canned
green pepper, finely chopped
1 1/2 cups lowfat milk

Soak beans in water. Add salt. Boil covered until almost done, about 1 hour. Add potato and onion; cook 30 minutes more. Mix flour with the margarine. Stir into bean mixture. Add tomatoes and green pepper. Cook over low heat 10 minutes, stirring constantly until thickened, then occasionally to avoid scorching. Stir in the milk. Heat to serving temperature. Serves 6.

Peppy Purple Borscht

1 tablespoon soft margarine
4 medium onions, chopped
4 medium potatoes, thinly sliced
1 cup beets, thinly sliced
1 stalk celery, chopped
3 cups cabbage, chopped
3/4 teaspoon caraway seeds

4 cups stock or water
1 teaspoon salt
1/4 teaspoon dill weed
4 teaspoons cider vinegar
4 teaspoons honey
1 cup tomato puree
3/4 cup plain yogurt, lowfat

Cook potatoes and beets in water until tender (save the water). Saute onions in soft margarine in a large pot. Add caraway seeds and salt. Cook until onions are tender. Add celery and cabbage. Add water from beets and potatoes. Cook covered until all the vegetables are tender. Add potatoes and beets, and all remaining ingredients except yogurt. Cover and simmer for about 30 minutes. Just before serving, add 1/2 cup yogurt. Garnish with remaining yogurt. Serves 6.

Souper Split Pea

2 cups dried split peas (1 pound)
3 quarts cold water
1 onion, chopped
3 stalks celery (with tops), chopped
    fine
2 carrots, chopped
salt and pepper to taste

1/4 teaspoon dried thyme
1/4 teaspooon dried marjoram
1 bay leaf
Dash of cayenne
2 cups potatoes, diced in 1/2 inch
    cubes

Soak peas in water overnight. (Quick-cooking dried peas and beans do not require overnight soaking.) Add onion, carrots, and celery. Heat to boil; cover and simmer approximately 1 hour, until peas are tender and liquid is partially cooked down. Add potatoes and continue to simmer for 30 minutes more. Dilute as desired with additional lowfat milk or water. Serves 8.

Main Dishes

Baked Split Peas

3 cups split peas, cooked
2 cups cooked brown rice
2 cups canned tomatoes
1/2 teaspoon salt

1/2 cup onion, chopped fine
oil
3/4 cup bread crumbs

Oil baking dish and make layers of the peas, rice, tomatoes and onion. Sprinkle with salt. Cover with oiled bread crumbs and bake at 400° for 20 minutes. Serve with tomato or cheese sauce. Serves 6-8.

Bean Bamboozle

3 cups cooked kidney, lima or
   garbanzo beans (1 cup dried)
2 cups canned or cooked tomatoes
2 onions, chopped
1 tablespoon vinegar

1/4 cup green pepper, chopped
1 tablespoon vegetable oil
1/2 teaspoon each—basil, oregano,
   tarragon, marjoram

Saute onions and pepper in oil. Add all other ingredients and simmer until thickened. Garnish with orange slice and serve with beet tops and whole wheat bread or brown rice. Serves 4-8.

Bean-Vegetable Casserole

1/2 cup dry garbanzo or other beans
2 cups stock
1 bay leaf
1 teaspoon basil
1 teaspoon sage
1/2-1 teaspoon salt

1 clove garlic, crushed
1/4 pound string beans, sliced
2 large tomatoes, sliced
1/3 cup grated cheese
10 peppercorns

Soak the beans overnight in the stock with bay leaf, basil, sage, pepper, and garlic. Cook the beans with seasoning until very tender, remove the peppercorns, and salt. (You may also remove the bay leaf and garlic.) In an oiled casserole alternate layers of the drained beans, string beans, tomatoes and cheese, ending with cheese. Bake at 350° for 30 minutes. Garnish with fresh parsley. Serves 4-8.

Blintzes

Blintz Batter:
3 eggs	1 tablespoon oil
1 cup milk or water	3/4 cup sifted flour
1/2 teaspoon salt	oil for frying

Beat the eggs, milk, salt and salad oil together. Stir in the flour. Heat a little oil in a 6'' skillet. Pour about 2 tablespoons of the batter into it, tilting the pan to coat the bottom. Use just enough batter to make a very thin pancake. Let the bottom brown, then carefully turn out onto a napkin, browned side up. Make the rest of the pancakes. Spread 1 heaping tablespoon of the filling along one side of the pancake. Turn opposite sides in and roll up like a jelly roll. Bake then in a 425° oven until browned. Makes about 18 blintzes. Serve dairy blintzes with sour cream or lowfat yogurt. Top with fresh fruit in season.

Filling for blintzes:
Cheese: 2 cups drained lowfat	
cottage cheese (2% fat)	1 egg yolk
cinnamon to taste	3/4 teaspoon salt

Beat the cheese, egg yolk, salt and cinnamon together.

Boston Baked Beans

2 cups dry pea (navy), pinto or	1/2 small onion
kidney beans	1/4 teaspoon cloves
7 cups water	1 teaspoon mustard
1 1/2 teaspoon salt	1/2 cup molasses

Wash beans. Put beans into water and boil for 2 minutes. Remove from heat. Cover and let stand for 1 hour. Add salt and cook slowly 1 hour. Chop onion and mix with cloves, mustard and molasses. Stir into beans. Put beans in baking pan. Add enough hot water to cover beans. Cover pan and bake at 350°F (moderate oven) 1 1/2 to 2 hours. Serves 6.

Cauliflower Marranca

1 pound mushrooms, sliced	1 large onion, chopped
juice of 1 lemon	1/4 teaspoon pepper
1 large head cauliflower (in flower	1 teaspoon basil
pieces)	1 1/2 to 3 cups raw brown rice or
3 cloves crushed garlic	millet
2 1/2 cups grated cheese of your choice	1 bunch chopped parsley

Cook grains in water. Saute vegetables in oil with lemon and spices. Combine everything. Bake covered for 1/2 hour at 350°. Serves 4.

Cheese Fondue

2 tablespoons butter or margarine
3 cups whole wheat bread cubes
 (5 slices)
1 cup shredded sharp cheddar
 cheese (1/4 pound)

1 cup lowfat milk
1/2 teaspoon salt
dash of pepper
1/8 teaspoon mustard
1 egg, beaten

Melt butter in skillet. Add bread crumbs; stir until lightly browned. Place in greased 1-quart baking dish in alternate layers with cheese. Mix rest of ingredients and pour over. Sprinkle with paprika. Set in pan of water (1 inch deep). Bake at 350° for 40 minutes. Serve hot. Serves 4.

Chicken with Fruit Sauce

1 broiler chicken, cut in serving
 pieces
2-3 tablespoons corn oil
Flour for dusting
1/4 teaspoon ground pepper
1/4 teaspoon salt
1/2 cup orange juice

1 tablespoon parsley, chopped
1 tablespoon honey
2 tablespoons slivered orange rind
1 cup seedless white grapes, halved
1/2 cup toasted walnuts
Salt, pepper to taste
Sliced orange for garnish

Dust chicken pieces with flour, salt and pepper. Heat oil in skillet. Brown chicken on both sides. Add orange juice, parsley and honey. Cover and simmer for 15 minutes. Add slivered orange rind and cook 10 minutes longer or until tender. Remove chicken to serving platter. Add grapes and walnuts to gravy and stir for two minutes. Pour over chicken and garnish with orange slices. Serve over cooked rice. Serves 4.

Chop Suey

1 cup celery, cut in thin strips
celery leaves, minced
1 minced garlic clove
1/2 cup sliced mushrooms
1 onion (sliced)
2 tablespoons vegetable oil
1 1/4 cups chicken stock or bouillon
1/2 to 1 pound bean sprouts

2 tablespoons soy sauce
1 tablespoon cornstarch
1/2 cup green pepper, cut in thin
 strips
2 cups cooked, cubed chicken
1 can (5 ounces) water chestnuts,
 drained, sliced

Gently cook celery, garlic, mushrooms, and onion in hot oil about 3 minutes. Add 1 cup of chicken stock; mix cornstarch with remaining stock. Blend into vegetable mixture with green pepper; cook just until thick. Add chicken, bean sprouts, water chestnuts and soy sauce; heat well but let vegetables remain crisp. Serve with hot rice and slivered toasted almonds. Serves 4.

Con Queso Rice

1 1/2 cups raw brown rice
  (cooked with salt and pepper)
3/4 pound shredded jack cheese
1 small can chiles, chopped
1/2 pound ricotta cheese, thinned
  slightly with lowfat milk or
  yogurt

3 cloves garlic, minced or pressed
1/2 cup grated cheddar cheese
1 large onion, chopped
1/2 cup dry black beans (blackeyed
  peas or kidney beans) cooked

Mix rice, beans, garlic, onion, chiles. Layer this mixture alternately in a greased casserole with jack cheese and ricotta (spreading evenly over casserole). End with rice mixture. Bake at 350°F for 1/2 hour. During last few minutes of baking, sprinkle grated cheese over the top. Serves 6.

Cottage Cheese Squares

1 cup raw brown rice, cooked
1/2 cup dry Pinto beans, cooked
  (or substitute other beans)
2 eggs
1 cup lowfat milk
2 cups lowfat cottage cheese
1/2 cup minced onion

1/2 teaspoon salt
3 tablespoons chopped fresh parsley
1 tablespoon chopped fresh rosemary
1 cup grated raw carrot
1 teaspoon oil

While the rice and beans are cooking—beat the eggs; beat in the milk, cottage cheese, salt, herbs, and grated carrot. In a small frying pan, saute the onion until it is very soft, but not brown. Stir the onions into the cottage cheese and egg mixture. Drain the cooked beans and stir them into the cottage cheese mixture along with the rice. Turn the whole mixture into an oiled 7" x 11" pan. Bake at 375°F with a pan of hot water on the lower oven shelf for about 25 minutes. When it is done, a knife inserted in the center will come out clean, and the top will have a thin light brown crust.

Cool the casserole for about 10 minutes, cut into squares and serve. You may also chill it completely and serve cold. Serves 8.

Dill-Deviled Eggs

6 hard-cooked eggs
4 to 5 tablespoons lowfat yogurt

4 to 5 tablespoons chopped fresh dill
salt and pepper

Peel the eggs, cut them in half, and empty the yolks into a bowl. Mash the yolks with the yogurt and dill, adding salt and pepper to your taste. Put this mixture back into the egg whites and sprinkle a little more dill on top. Serve chilled. Serves 6.

Hopping John

1 pound blackeyed peas
2 quarts boiling water
1 onion, chopped
1 tablespoon corn oil
3/4 cup chopped celery

1 crushed garlic clove
1 bay leaf
Salt and pepper to taste
Crushed red peppers
1 cup raw rice, cooked

Wash the blackeyed peas, soak overnight in cold water; or boil them for 2 minutes and soak 1 hour or longer (or use the quick cooking variety). Drain

228

well. Put the peas in a large pot, add the boiling water, onion, celery, oil and seasonings. Simmer, covered, for about 2 hours, or until peas are very soft, adding water as needed. Taste and season as desired. Add the cooked rice to the cooked peas in the pot. Simmer gently until all liquid is absorbed. Serves 6.

Individual Muffin Pizzas

Toast halves of bagels or English muffins, or slices of whole wheat bread under broiler. Cover each with tomato slices, tomato paste, onion rings. Sprinkle with pepper and oregano. Top with a slice of part-skimmed mozzarella or lowfat cottage cheese and a mushroom cap. Return to broiler until cheese melts and bubbles. Serve hot.

Italian-Style Cheese Noodle Casserole

8 ounces wide whole wheat noodles
20 ounces tomato sauce
2 cups lowfat cottage cheese
1/2 teaspoon dried crushed basil
1/2 teaspoon salt

1/4 cup finely diced onions
1/2 pound cheddar or Wisconsin
  Brick cheese, grated
1/2 cup bread crumbs
1/4 cup grated Parmesan or Romano
  cheese

Cook noodles in boiling salted water; rinse and drain. Combine tomato sauce, cottage cheese, basil, salt and onion; blend well. Arrange alternate layers of noodles, cheese, and cause in a 3 quart carrerole. Top with crumbs mixed with grated Parmesan cheese. Bake in a 350-375° oven for approximately 25 minutes or until hot. Garnish with fresh parsley. Serves 8.

Lentil Loaf

1 cup lentils
1/2 cup barley
4 cups water
1 teaspoon salt
1 cup bread crumbs

1 clove garlic, minced
1 medium onion, minced
1 rib celery, sliced thinly
2 eggs, beaten
1/8 teaspoon nutmeg

Add lentils and barley to boiling salted water. Allow to boil for a minute, then reduce heat and simmer with lid ajar for about 40 minutes or until most of the water is absorbed. Remove from heat. Add bread crumbs along with remaining ingredients and mix well. Place mixture in a well oiled 9x5x3 inch loaf pan and bake at 350° for 35 minutes. Allow to cool for 15-20 minutes before inverting over a platter to serve. Serves 6-8.

Lentil-Mushroom Stew

1 1/2 quarts stock or water
2 cups lentils, washed
1 onion, sliced and chopped
1/2 pound mushrooms, sliced
1/2 teaspoon salt

2 stalks celery and tops, chopped
2 carrots, sliced
1 can stewed tomatoes
2 tablespoons oil
2 tablespoons vinegar

Bring stock to a boil and slowly add lentils. Reduce to a simmer and cook 1 hour. Saute onion, mushrooms, and basil in oil. Set aside. Combine all ingredients except vinegar and seasonings; cook at least 1 more hour, or until lentils are tender. Add vinegar before serving. Add salt and pepper to taste. Serves 4 well.

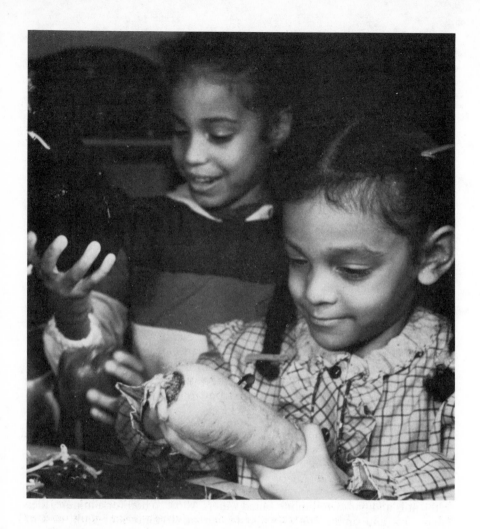

Mediterranean Ratatouille

2 onions, sliced
1 tablespoon oil
2 small eggplants (about one pound each), peeled and cubed
5 tomatoes, or 2 cups canned tomatoes, chopped
2 tablespoons parsley

1 garlic clove, minced
2 small zucchini, thinly sliced
2 green peppers, cut into 1 inch strips
1 tablespoon basil
1/2 teaspoon salt
1/4 teaspoon pepper

Using a large, heavy skillet, saute onions and garlic in 1 tablespoon of olive oil (or a little water) for 5 minutes. Add zucchini, eggplant, and green pepper to skillet, adding more oil or water if needed. Stir gently, but thoroughly. Saute mixture for 5-10 minutes. Stir in the fresh or canned tomatoes, basil, parsley, salt and pepper. Reduce heat, cover skillet tightly, and continue to simmer for 15 minutes longer. Serve immediately. Try a layer of ricotta, cheddar or lowfat cottage cheese on top. Serves 8-10.

Mexican Enchiladas

Tortillas:

1 cup whole wheat flour
1/2 cup corn meal
1/4 teaspoon salt

1 egg
1 1/2 cups cold water

Combine ingredients in bowl. Beat with rotary beater until smooth. Spoon 1 tablespoon butter on a moderately hot ungreased griddle to make a very thin 6" pancake. Turn tortillas when edges begin to look dry, not brown. Cook other side; keep warm in covered pan. Makes 12 Tortillas.

Tortilla Filling:

2 cups grated sharp Cheddar cheese
1 cup minced onion

1 cup mashed, cooked beans
1/2 teaspoon salt

Mix ingredients thoroughly.

Enchiladas Sauce:

2 tablespoons minced onion
2 tablespoons corn oil
1 tablespoon flour, enriched
1 can (1 pound, 4 ounces)
    tomatoes, drained

2 teaspoon chili powder
1 teaspoon salt
1/4 teaspoon Tabasco

Brown onion in hot oil. Stir in flour. Then stir in rest of ingredients. Add about 1/2 cup tomato juice (drained from tomatoes) to make a sauce of medium thickness. Let simmer until thickened.

Dip tortillas into Enchiladas Sauce (above). Place a large spoonful of Tortilla Filling (above) on each and roll up. Arrange in serving dish or baking dish. Cover with hot sauce and sprinkle with remaining filling. Serve at once or re-heat before serving at 375°. Serves 6.

Note: Enchiladas fit well in an 11" x 7 1/2" x 1 1/2" baking dish or 13" x 9 1/2" x 2" pan. They may be kept hot in the oven for some time if covered with aluminum foil.

Mexican Grains

1 cup raw brown rice plus 3/4 cup
    raw bulgur, cooked together in 4
    cups of water
2/3 cup dry soybeans, cooked
Oil as needed
1 tablespoon green chilis, diced
1 small can corn

1/2 pound string beans, sliced into
    2" pieces
1 teaspoon chili powder (to taste)
Dash hot sauce
Salt and pepper
1 can (16 ounces) stewed tomatoes

Heat oil in heavy pot or skillet. Add the green chilis and saute until tender. To the chilis, add the sliced string beans and continue sauteeing while adding in the chili powder, hot sauce, and salt and pepper. Mix in the stewed tomatoes, corn, grains, and soybeans. Simmer for about 15 minutes. Serves 8-10.

Mexican Pan Bread

1/2 cup dry beans, cooked with extra water (a dark bean such as kidney or black bean makes the dish colorful)
3/4 cup water or vegetable stock
1 onion, chopped
1 egg, beaten
1 cup cornmeal
1 teaspoon chili powder or more to taste
1/2 teaspoon cumin
1/4 teaspoon salt
1/3 cup grated cheese
1 clove garlic, minced
2 teaspoon baking powder

Saute onion and garlic in a small heavy skillet. Mix together all remaining ingredients except for the cheese. Pour this mixture into the skillet and stir to mix well. Sprinkle grated cheese on top and bake at 350° for about 15 minutes. A quick delicious meal—good with soup and salad. Serves 6-8.

Mushroom Curry

1-2 tablespoons oil
1/2 pound fresh mushrooms— chop the stems and leave the caps whole
1 onion, minced
1 tablespoon curry powder
2 apples, chopped fine (chop one of the apples just before serving)
salt
paprika
2 2/3 cup lowfat yogurt
2 cups raw brown rice, cooked and hot OR 1 1/2 cups raw bulgur wheat, cooked and hot

Saute the mushroom caps in oil for about 5 minutes, until they just absorb the oil and are slightly brown. Set them aside in a small bowl. Add more oil to the pan and saute the onion and curry powder until the onion is almost transparent. Add one chopped apple and the mushroom stems; continue sauteeing until the onion is transparent. Don't let the apple get too mushy. Remove from the heat and stir in paprika, salt to taste, and the yogurt.

To assemble the dish: Place the cooked grain in a 2 or 2 1/2 quart casserole. Spread the mushroom-yogurt sauce evenly over the grain. Then arrange the mushroom caps on the top. Sprinkle with more paprika. Bake the casserole at 350°F until the sauce is firm. Sprinkle the freshly chopped apple over the top just before serving. Serves 8.

Noodle Kugel

3 eggs
1 3/4 cups plain lowfat yogurt
2 teaspoons cinnamon
2 apples (cooking kind, not Delicious) or 2 fresh peaches, sliced
1 1/2 cups lowfat cottage cheese
1/2 teaspoon vanilla
1/4 cup honey or brown sugar
Scant 1/2 teaspoon salt
4 cups (raw) wide, flat egg noodles

Boil noodles in salted water until tender (not soft); drain. Combine remaining ingredients. Spread into buttered oblong baking pan (9" x 13"). Top with mixture of 1 cup bread crumbs and 1 teaspoon of cinnamon. Bake uncovered for 35 minutes at 375°. Serves 8.

Pinto Bean Pie

1, 9 or 10 inch whole wheat pie
 shell, partially cooked
2 large onions, chopped
1 tablespoon honey

1 tablespoon corn oil
2 cups well-cooked beans
1/4 teaspoon salt
2-3 tablespoons cinnamon

Saute onions in oil until very soft. Drain and blend beans, onions, salt, and cinnamon until smooth in a blender. Pour all into the partly cooked pie shell. For variety, omit beans and honey and add 2 cups cooked and mashed sweet potato, butternut squash or carrots. Sprinkle with topping. Bake about 15 minutes at 350°.

Quick Macaroni

8 ounces whole wheat macaroni
6-8 ounces sharp Cheddar cheese
 or lowfat cottage cheese
1/8 teaspoon pepper

1 1/2 cups tomato sauce
2 cups sliced mushrooms
1/2 cup chopped celery
1 cup chopped broccoli

Cook macaroni in boiling water for about 15 minutes, drain. Add heated tomato sauce, shredded cheese, sliced mushrooms, celery, and broccoli. Stir. Serve garnished with celery leaves.

Roman Rice and Beans

1 1/2 cup dried pea beans (cook
 until tender in 2 quarts water)
2 large onions, finely chopped
2 garlic cloves, crushed
1-2 carrots, finely chopped
1 stalk celery, chopped (optional)
2/3 cup parsley, chopped
5-6 teaspoons dried basil

1 teaspoon dried oregano
2 large tomatoes, coarsely chopped
Salt and pepper to taste
4 cups raw brown rice, cooked
1/4 cup margarine
1 cup grated cheese (Parmesan or
 jack)
1 tablespoon oil

Saute onions, garlic, carrots, celery, parsley, basil and oregano in oil until onion is golden. Add tomatoes, salt, and pepper, and cooked beans. Add margarine and cheese to cooked rice. Then add first mixture. Garnish with more parsley and more grated cheese. Serves 8-10.

Soy Burgers

1 can (15 1/2 ounces) soybeans,
 drained and rinsed, or 2 cups
 cooked soybeans
2 eggs, lightly beaten
1 teaspoon basil, oregano, sage
1 tomato, skinned and put
 through an electric blender until
 smooth

1 small onion, finely grated or
 chopped
1 cup wheat germ
1 tablespoon tamari (soy sauce)
1 teaspoon thyme

Preheat the oven to 350°. Mash the soybeans with a potato masher. In a large bowl, combine all the ingredients. Using a small ice cream scoop, measure out portions of mixture onto a lightly oiled baking sheet. Flatten each scoop slightly. Bake 25 minutes, turn and bake 15 minutes longer. Serves 4.

Spinach Lasagna

1 pound whole wheat lasagna
  noodles

Filling:
2 bunches spinach, finely chopped
2 tablespoons Parmesan cheese
1 cup lowfat cottage cheese (1/2
  pound)
1/4 teaspoon nutmeg

Sauce:
2 cups tomato sauce
2 cloves garlic, minced and sauteed
1/2 cup onions, chopped and sauteed
1/2 teaspoon basil
Add pepper to taste

Steam spinach until it is quite limp, but not mushy. To do this place washed spinach in a pan which has a tight-fitting cover and cook over low heat about 7 minutes. Mix the spinach with the cheese, nutmeg, and pepper. Cook noodles in boiling water for 10 minutes. Remove. Coat each noodle with 2 to 3 tablespoons of the mixture along its entire length, roll up, turn on end so that you see the spiral, and place in a shallow baking pan. Mix all of the sauce ingredients together and pour over rolled-up noodles. Bake at 350°F. for 20 minutes. (You can substitute your favorite tomato sauce recipe.) Serves 4.

Stuffed Peppers

6 green peppers
3/4 cup brown rice
1 3/4 cups water
1 teaspoon salt
1 tablespoon oil

1 medium onion, minced
1/4 cup sesame seeds
1 1/2 cups chopped tomato
1/4 teaspoon basil
1 tablespoon soy sauce

Wash rice, then bring to a boil with water and salt. Allow to boil for a minute, reduce heat and simmer, covered, for 40-45 minutes. Place a frying pan on medium heat and add oil. When oil is hot add onion; stir for a few minutes until transparent, add sesame seeds and stir a few minutes more. Add tomato and basil and simmer about 5 minutes. If necessary, add a small amount of water to keep from burning. Slice tops off peppers and remove pulp and seeds. When rice is done, mix well with vegetables and soy sauce; then fill each pepper with this mixture. Sprinkle a bit of grated cheese on top if desired and replace pepper tops. Steam for about 20 minutes until peppers are tender; in a vegetable steamer, or by placing in the bottom of a covered pot with a little water and simmering over low heat.

Stir-Fry Frenzy

1-2 teaspoons sesame or peanut oil
3 or more cloves garlic, mashed
1 tablespoon sesame seeds
2 stalks broccoli, slices and flower-
    ettes
1 handful mushrooms, sliced in
    thick slices
1 green pepper, diced

2 medium onions, sliced
1/2 teaspoon dried rosemary,
    crushed
2 large carrots, sliced diagonally
Cauliflowerettes
1 handful spinach leaves
Soy sauce

Optional: Strips of meat or chicken; chunks of tofu; nuts of any kind; pine-apple chunks

Stir-fry the onions, garlic, rosemary and sesame seeds in oil, until the onions start to brown. Stir in the hard vegetables (carrots, broccoli, cauliflower). Put the cover on the pan and cook until the vegetables are about half done, about 6 minutes. Add soy sauce to keep everything from sticking. Add mush-rooms. Stir and cook about 4 minutes. Add the spinach leaves and green pepper. As soon as these are just warm, slightly wilted, serve over the grains. Serves 4.

For variation, mix yogurt with grated mild cheese and minced herbs, smooth over vegetables and heat in the oven.

Other Vegetables for Stir-Fry

Hard Vegetables (12-15 minutes)	Medium Vegetables (8-10 minutes)	Soft Vegetables (3-4 minutes)
Green beans	Asparagus	Spinach
Celery	Mushrooms	Chinese cabbage
Carrots	Snow peas	Beet greens
Broccoli	Green peas	Swiss chard
Cabbage	Zucchini	Fresh basil
Cauliflower	Yellow summer squash	Fresh parsley
Kale	Eggplant	Scallions
Bok choy	Radishes	Sprouts
Green tomatoes	Corn	Green peppers
Potatoes	Red tomatoes	
Plantains		

Sukiyaki

1 pound round steak
1/2 pound mushrooms, thinly sliced
1 bunch green onions, cut in
    1 1/2 inch lengths
3 stalks celery, sliced
2 large onions, thinly sliced

1 teaspoon soy sauce
1 can (8 ounces) bamboo shoots,
3 tablespoons water
3 cups raw spinach leaves
3 cups cooked rice, brown

Cut round steak in pieces 2 x 1/2 inches and brown. Add all ingredients ex-cept spinach and rice. Simmer until vegetables are tender, about 10 minutes. Add spinach; cook five minutes. Serve on rice. Serves 4.

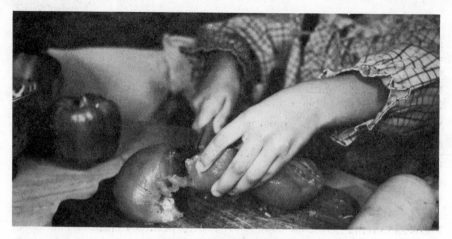

Swiss Vegetable Bake

1 tablespoon oil
2 cups onions, sliced
3 stalks sliced broccoli
1/2 pound mushrooms, sliced
1/2 cup watercress or parsley, chopped
3 cups cooked brown rice

1 clove garlic, minced
1 1/2 teaspoons paprika
1 teaspoon salt
1/2 teaspoon black pepper
1/4 teaspoon ground ginger
1 pound Swiss cheese, coarsely grated

Heat a large skillet. Add oil and saute the onions, broccoli, mushrooms, and watercress or parsley. Add garlic, paprika, salt, pepper and a little ginger to taste. Layer the brown rice, vegetables, and grated Swiss cheese in a shallow casserole. Repeat layers. If it seems dry, sprinkle with a cup vegetable stock or juice before adding last layer of cheese. Bake for 20-25 minutes at 350°. Garnish with tomato wedges, chopped parsley or chopped watercress.

Sweet-and-Sour Stuffed Cabbage

12 whole cabbage leaves, steamed until limp
1 1/4 cups raw brown rice and
2 tablespoons soy grits, cooked together, plus 1/2 teaspoon salt

toasted sunflower seeds
1 scant tablespoon caraway seed
1/2 cup raisins

Saute:

1 tablespoon oil
1 onion, chopped

Sauce:

1 15 ounce can tomato sauce with
1 tablespoon lemon juice and
1 teaspoon brown sugar (more to taste)

Combine rice mixture with sauteed ingredients. Add enough tomato sauce to moisten mixture. Place about 3 tablespoons of this filling on each cabbage leaf and roll up, securing with a toothpick if necessary. Place the rolls in a skillet and pour the remaining tomato sauce over them. Cover and cook about 15 minutes or until cabbage is quite tender. Top with lowfat yogurt. Serves 4.

Tamale Pie

1 large onion, chopped
1/2 pound lean ground beef
1 large can pear tomatoes
1 can (17 ounces) creamed corn
1 can (9 ounces) pitted black olives

1 1/2 teaspoon chili powder
1 1/2 cups yellow corn meal
2 eggs
1 cup lowfat milk

Mix together beef, onions, tomatoes, corn, olives, salt and chili powder. Mix together corn meal, eggs and milk. Combine the mixtures, add sauteed onions and bake in large casserole at 350° for one hour. Serves 4-6.

Tomato Rarebit

2 tablespoons margarine
4 tablespoons whole wheat flour
1 cup grated sharp cheddar
   cheese

1/2 teaspoon soy sauce
2 cups tomato juice

Melt margarine in sauce pan. Add next 3 ingredients, blending well. Stir in tomato juice, cooking and stirring until thick. Add cheese and remove from heat when cheese is melted. Serve over toast. Serves 4-6.

Tuna and Corn Casserole

2 cans (6 1/2 or 7 ounce each) tuna
   (preferably canned in water)
1/2 cup chopped onion
1/4 cup chopped green pepper
1 tablespoon oil
1 package (8 ounces) macaroni,
   whole wheat

1 can (1 pound 4 ounces) cream-
   style corn
3/4 cup lowfat milk
pepper
paprika

Drain tuna; break into large pieces. Cook onion and green pepper in oil until tender. Cook macaroni as directed on package; drain. Combine all ingredients except paprika. Place in a well greased, 2-quart casserole. Sprinkle with paprika. Bake in a moderate oven, 350°F., for 50 minutes. Serves 6.

Tuna and Rice Croquettes

1 cup cooked brown rice
1 can (6 1/2 ounces) tuna,
   (preferably canned in water)
1 egg, separated
2 tablespoons minced onion

1 teaspoon lemon juice
1/2 teaspoon salt
1/8 teaspoon pepper
3/4 cup whole wheat bread crumbs

Combine slightly beaten egg yolk with flaked tuna. Add rice and seasonings; chill. Just before shaping, fold in stiffly beaten egg white. Shape into 8 patties or cones. Roll in bread crumbs. Bake in over 350°F. for 30 minutes. Serve hot with tomato or cheese sauce. Serves 4.

Vegie Burgers

1 cup millet
1 tablespoon oil
1/8 teaspoon cayenne (red pepper)
3 cups boiling water
1 teaspoon salt
3/4 cup grated carrot

3/4 cup minced onion
1/2 cup minced parsley
1/2 cup whole wheat flour
1/4 cup soy flour
1/4 cup soy flour oil for frying

Place a large pot on medium heat and add oil. When oil is hot add millet and cayenne and stir for 2-3 minutes until millet gives off a nutlike fragrance. Add boiling salted water and reduce heat to simmer. Simmer, covered, for 35-40 minutes, adding vegetables 5 minutes before done. Add flours to millet and vegetables, mixing well to avoid lumps. Let mixture sit for 15-20 minutes until cool enough to handle. Heat oil about 1/8 inch deep in a frying pan on medium-low heat. Form millet mixture into thick patties with hands, or press into shape with a pancake turner. Fry for 3-4 minutes on each side or until crisp and lightly browned. Serve with soy sauce or your favorite sauce or gravy. Makes 18-20 burgers.

Winter Squash or Pumpkin Pie

1 uncooked 9-inch whole wheat
  pie shell
1 cup lowfat milk
1 teaspoon tamari (soy sauce)
3 cloves garlic, minced
1-2 tablespoons oil

3 cups cooked winter squash or
  pumpkin
1/2 onion, chopped
2 eggs, beaten
4 tablespoons chopped parsley

Mix all the filling ingredients together until fairly smooth. Pour into the pie shell. Bake 45 minutes at 375° or until the pie is firm in the center. Serves 6.

Breads, Cereals and Pancakes

BREADS

Basic Yeast Bread

1/4 cup (1/8 pound) butter,
  margarine, or corn oil
1/4 cup molasses
1 package yeast, active dry or
  compressed
1 egg, slightly beaten
About 4 cups whole wheat flour

1 teaspoon salt
1 cup lowfat milk, scalded and
  cooled to lukewarm
1/4 cup warm water (lukewarm for
  compressed yeast)
Softened butter

Place the butter, salt, and sugar in a large bowl; add the lukewarm milk, stirring to dissolve the sugar and salt and to melt the butter. Soften the yeast in the warm water and add, along with the beaten egg, to the milk mixture. Stir in 3 1/2 cups of the flour, 1 cup at a time, beating vigorously to blend. Scrape dough from the sides of the bowl and brush the top of the dough and the sides of the bowl with softened butter. Cover dough and let rise in a warm place about 2 hours, or until almost doubled in bulk. Then turn out on a well-floured board and knead lightly, adding flour until the dough is no longer sticky (do not use more than 1/4 to 1/2 cup flour on the board). Shape and bake. Bake loaves for 45 minutes at 350°. Bake rolls 10-12 minutes at 425°.

Variations

Take dough the size of a loaf of bread. Roll out with rolling pin in rectangular shape 10 x 24 inches and 1/4 inch thick. Spread with any of the fillings below. Roll up like a jelly roll. Slice into about 3/4 inch slices. Place on greased pie plate or rectangular pans, cover. Let rise. Bake.

1. *Cheese-Nut Rolls*—Mix 1 cup dry, lowfat cottage cheese (pot cheese) with 1/4 cup chopped walnuts and 1/2 teaspoon cinnamon.

2. *Apple and Raisin Rolls*—1 cup chopped apples, 1/4 cup nuts, 1/4 cup raisins, 1/2 teaspoon nutmeg mixed together.

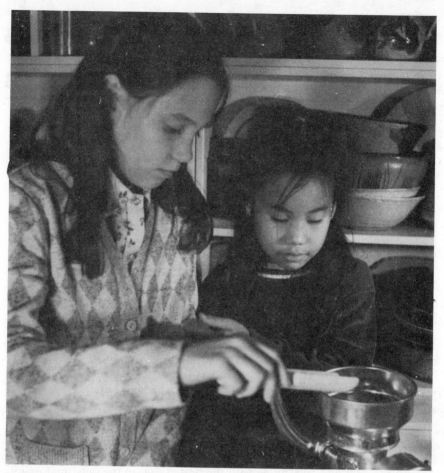

3. *Dates and Orange Rolls*—Mix 1 cup dates with 1/2 cup concentrated thawed frozen orange juice. Cook until dates are soft. Cook to lukewarm.

4. *Cranberry-Raisin Rolls*—Combine 1 cup cranberries, 1/2 cup raisins, and 2 tablespoons of honey or brown sugar.

5. *Peaches and Nut Rolls*—Combine 1 cup fresh sliced peaches, 1/4 cup walnuts, 1/2 teaspoon nutmeg and 2 tablespoons brown sugar.

6. *Blueberry-Raisin Rolls*—Combine 1 cup blueberries, 1/2 cup raisins, and 1/2 teaspoon cinnamon.

7. *Easter Bread*—Add 1/2 cup raisins and 1/2 cup nuts to bread dough. Bake in clean greased metal pails. (Paint stores carry them—very inexpensive). Or use 3 pound coffee cans. The bread rises high to symbolize rising from death to new life.

8. *Irish Barmbrack Bread*—The Irish serve this bread for Halloween to predict the fortune for the coming year. A ring (to symbolize an approaching marriage), a coin (wealth), and a button (many blessings) are put into the loaf. Wrap them in foil. 3/4 cup each raisins and currants, grated rind of a lemon and orange are added to the dough. Shape dough into large round loaves, cover, let rise. Bake.

Bountiful Whole Wheat Yeast Bread*
(2 loaves)

I.

3 cups lukewarm water (85°-100°F.)
   (can substitute 2 cups fresh apple juice—85°-100°F.)
1 package fresh cake yeast or 1 package dry yeast
1 teaspoon sugar (for "proofing" yeast)
1/3 cup sweetening (honey, molasses, brown sugar)
1 package dry milk or (4 to 5 tablespoons)
4 1/2 cups whole wheat flour *or* (substitute the following to total 4 1/2 cups):
   1/2 cup soy flour
   1/2 cup wheat germ
   1/2 cup bran
   1/2 cup rolled oats
   1 1/2 cups unbleached white flour

II.

1 1/4 tablespoon salt
1/2 cup corn or safflower oil
4 cups additional whole wheat flour

1/2 cup sunflower seeds (optional)
1/2 cup raisins (optional)
1/4 cup walnuts (optional)

Proof yeast—dissolve yeast in water (1/4 cup plus 1 teaspoon sugar). When yeast begins to bubble, it is proofed (active).

In a large mixing bowl, put 2 3/4 cups water (part apple juice). Add 1 package dry milk powder. Add sweetener (molasses preferred). Stir in dissolved (proofed) yeast. Stir in the 4 1/2 cups flour mixture: soy flour, wheat germ, bran, rolled oats, unbleached flour, whole wheat flour.

Add salt and oil. (Blend in). Fold in 4 cups of whole wheat flour. (Additional). Add nuts, raisins, and knead until dough is smooth and elastic. More flour may be needed if dough is sticky.

Knead on floured board, using more flour if needed until dough is smooth. Oil dough to prevent from drying. Let rise 50 minutes. (double in size). Punch down. Let rise 40 minutes. Shape into loaves, put into oiled pans. Let rise 20 minutes. Brush surface with beaten egg-wash. Sprinkle with sesame seeds (Black Russian seeds are delicious.) Bake in 350°F oven for 45-55 minutes. Remove from pan and let cool on rack.

Oatmeal Bread

1 envelope yeast
1/4 cup lukewarm water
1/3 cup brown sugar
2 cups scalding milk or water

2 cups rolled oats
2 tablespoons oil
4 cups whole wheat flour
1 tablespoon salt

Put the yeast, lukewarm water, and sugar in a small bowl, and let stand until frothy. Pour the scalding liquid over the oats and oil and let it stand until it is lukewarm. Sift the flour with the salt. Combine the yeast, oats and 1 cup of the flour and beat well. Set the bowl in a dishpan of quite warm water, cover

*Courtesy of Hedda Batwin

with a tea towel and let the dough rise until light. Push down and add the rest of the flour. If the dough is too heavy to be resilient add a very small amount of warm water.

Knead it on a floured board until light. Let it rise again in a pan of warm water, covered, until it doubles. Push down again and put the dough in two oiled bread pans to rise. When the dough is at the top of the pans put it in a 400°F. oven for 20 minutes, turn down the heat to 350°F. and bake 25 minutes more. A pan of hot water set on the oven floor while the bread is baking makes a chewy brown crust. When adding water or milk to dough containing cereals, be careful not to add too much or the bread will sink in the middle when baked.

Rye Bread

1 tablespoon dry yeast
1 1/2 cups warm water
1/4 cup molasses
3 to 3 1/2 cups whole wheat flour
1 cup rye flour

1 teaspoon salt
2 tablespoons oil
1/2 tablespoon caraway seeds, whole
 or ground

Dissolve yeast in warm water and add sweetener. Let sit for 5 minutes, then add 2 cups whole wheat flour and beat well to form a smooth, thick, elastic batter. Let sit for about 1 hour until light and foamy. Mix in salt, oil, and caraway. Add the rye flour and some of the remaining wholewheat flour and begin to knead.

Knead well, adding more flour a small amount at a time until dough is smooth and elastic. The exact amount of flour to be used will vary slightly each time. Let rise for 45 minutes—1 hour, then punch down, knead for a few minutes. Shape into a loaf and place in a lightly-oiled bread pan. Let rise in the pan for about 45 minutes, until not quite doubled in bulk. Preheat oven to 350° while rising. Bake for about 1 hour; remove from pan at once and cool before slicing.

Note: Rye flour is best combined with other flour(s) for bread baking. It has little gluten and does not rise well if used alone.

Two-Hour Bread

Mix in bowl:

3 cups warm water
3 tablespoons yeast
1/3 cup honey or molasses
3 tablespoons oil

Add:

6 1/2 cups whole wheat flour
1 tablespoon salt
1 cup powdered milk

Let rise in warm place covered—15 minutes. After resting, knead well for 10 minutes. Sprinkle flour on table and hands often. Fill pans (greased) 2/3 full. Let rise 15 minutes in warm place. Bake in 375° pre-heated oven 20-30 minutes. Makes 2 loaves.

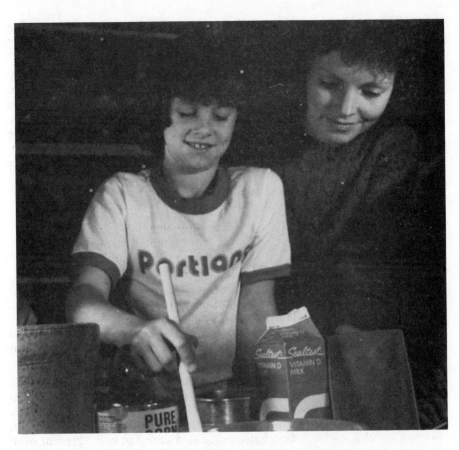

Blueberry Muffins

2 cups whole wheat flour
1/4 cup sugar
1 cup lowfat milk, approximately
2 eggs, lightly beaten

1/2 teaspoon salt
1 tablespoon baking powder
1/4 cup oil
1 cup blueberries

Preheat the oven to 400°. In a mixing bowl, combine the flour, salt, sugar, baking powder. Stir in enough milk to make a stiff dough. Stir in the oil, eggs and blueberries. Spoon into oiled muffin tins so that they are two-thirds full. Bake 30 minutes or until done. About one dozen two-inch muffins.

Bran Muffins

1 egg, beaten
1 1/2 cup lowfat milk
1/4 cup oil
1 cup bran
1/4 cup honey

1 cup flour, whole wheat
2 teaspoons baking powder
1/4 cup molasses
1/4 teaspoon salt
1/2 cup raisins

Mix egg, milk, oil and bran in bowl. Let stand 10 minutes. Add the dry ingredients, stirring just enough to dampen flour. Spoon into greased muffin tins. Bake at 400° about 25 minutes. Makes 12.

Brown Rice and Whole Wheat Muffins

1 1/4 cups whole wheat flour
1/2 teaspoon salt
1 cup cold (not chilled) cooked
   brown rice
2/3 cup lowfat milk

2 teaspoons baking powder
2 tablespoons molasses
1/4 cup oil
2 eggs, lightly beaten

Preheat the oven to 425°. In a bowl, combine the flour, baking powder, and salt; mix well. Add the rice, oil, eggs, milk and molasses. Spoon mixture into oiled and floured muffin tins. Bake 15 to 20 minutes or until done. One dozen medium-size muffins. Note: The rice gives a crunchy texture to the muffins.

Corn Bread

1 cup cornmeal
1 cup whole wheat flour
2 teaspoons baking powder
1/2 teaspoon baking soda
1/4 cup honey

1/4 teaspoon salt
1 egg, beaten
1 cup buttermilk or lowfat yogurt
3 tablespoons oil

Stir together all of the dry ingredients in a large bowl. Stir the liquid ingredients together in a separate bowl and then stir them into the dry ingredients, mixing only enough to combine the ingredients thoroughly. Less mixing will make a more tender bread. Pour the batter into an oiled 9" x 9" pan and bake at 350°F for 40 to 50 minutes. The top will spring back when the bread is done and a tester should come out clean but moist (not uncooked batter) but it may be moister than normally expected.

This cornbread is most delicious when eaten warm with a small amount of honey, lowfat yogurt or molasses.

Crusty Popover

3 eggs
1/2 cup instant nonfat dry milk
1 cup water
6-7 buttered custard cups

2 tablespoons melted margarine
1/2 teaspoon salt
1 cup sifted flour, whole wheat

Beat eggs until light, add instant nonfat dry milk, water, melted butter and salt. Blend well. Gradually beat in flour. Set cups well apart in cake pan. Fill each cup 2/3 full of batter. Bake 50-60 minutes at 400° or until popovers are high, crusty and well browned. Remove from cups at once and cut slit inside of each to allow steam to escape. Serve hot.

Oatmeal Muffins

1 cup whole wheat flour
1/4 cup molasses
3 teaspoons baking powder
1/2 cup raisins
3 teaspoons oil

1/2 teaspoon salt
1 cup rolled oats
1 slightly beaten egg
1 cup milk

Mix thoroughly flour, salt, oats, raisins and baking powder. Then mix egg, molasses, milk and oil and combine with dry ingredients. Stir enough just to moisten (fill a 12-cup greased muffin pan or medium-sized loaf pan 2/3 full). Bake at 425° about 15 minutes (20-25 minutes for loaf.)

Rieska

1 7/8 cups whole wheat or rye flour	1/2 teaspoon salt
2 teaspoons sugar	2 teaspoons baking powder
1 cup undiluted evaporated milk	1 tablespoon margarine, melted

In a bowl combine the flour with the salt, sugar, and baking powder. Stir in the milk and the melted butter or margarine until a smooth dough forms. Turn the dough out onto a well-oiled cookie sheet, dust your hands lightly with flour and pat the dough out to make a circle about 14 inches in diameter and 1/2 inch thick.

Prick all over with a fork, and bake in a very hot oven (450°) for 10 minutes or until lightly browned. Serve immediately cut in pie-shaped wedges and spread with butter. Makes 8-10 pieces. Rieska is a traditional Finland or Lapland favorite.

Scottish Scones

1 7/8 cups whole wheat flour	2 eggs (reserve small amount of white
4 teaspoons baking powder	to brush tops)
1/2 teaspoon salt	1/3 cup lowfat milk
2 tablespoons sugar	1/2 cup raisins (optional)
4 tablespoons butter or margarine	

Sift dry ingredients into bowl. Cut in butter or margarine. Beat eggs well, add milk and stir carefully into a well in center of flour mixture, until all is dampened. Then stir vigorously for a few seconds. Turn out on lightly floured board; knead 30 seconds. Roll 1/2 inch thick, cut in triangles or diamond shape. Place on greased baking sheet. Brush tops with the reserved egg white, slightly beaten, sprinkle with sugar. Bake in hot oven (450°F) 12 minutes, or until browned. For variety, add grated lemon rind or orange rind to sugar sprinkled on top.

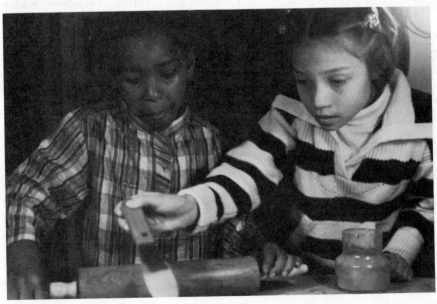

Spoon Bread

3 cups lowfat milk
3/4 teaspoon salt
1 tablespoon sugar
3 eggs, separated

1 cup yellow corn meal
1 teaspoon baking powder
2 tablespoons oil

Preheat the oven to 350°. Heat two cups of the milk in a saucepan. When milk begins to simmer, add the corn meal and continue to cook, stirring until mixture is thick. Remove from the heat and add salt, baking powder, sugar, oil and remaining cup of milk. Beat the egg yolks lightly and add to corn meal mixture. Beat the eggs whites until stiff but not dry and fold into corn meal mixture. Turn into a buttered two-quart souffle dish and bake one hour or until well puffed and brown on top. Serve by the spoonful directly from the dish and top with butter. Serves 8.

Whole Wheat Muffins

2 cups whole wheat flour
2 teaspoons baking powder
1/4 teaspoon salt
1 egg, beaten

1/4 cup oil
1/4 cup honey or molasses
1 1/2 cup low fat milk

Combine all dry ingredients. Combine liquid ingredients. Fold quickly liquid and dry together, just until flour is moistened. Spoon into muffin tin. Bake at 400°F. for about 20 minutes.

Variations

1. substitute 1 cup apple sauce for 1 cup of the milk
2. add raisins and/or chopped nuts
3. add spices such as cinnamon, nutmeg, etc.
4. combine all or parts of the first three variations
5. substitute 1 1/2 cup buttermilk for milk, and substitute 1 teaspoon baking powder and 3/4 teaspoon baking soda for 2 teaspoons baking powder.

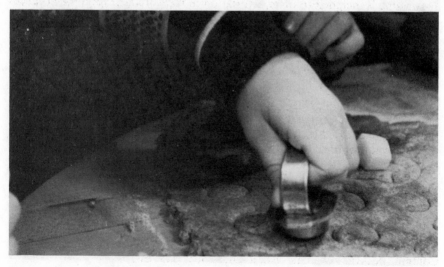

CEREALS

Coldstuff for Warm Mornings

3 cups quick oats
1 1/2 cups raw or toasted wheat germ
1 (8 ounces) package dried apricots,
   minced

3 cups rolled wheat or wheat flakes
2 cups raisins
1/2-1 cup brown sugar (optional)
1 cup chopped nuts

Mix everything together and store in jars in the refrigerator. You may substitute or add any dried fruits or nuts available. Any flaked grain may be used, such as bran, rye, etc. Familia is to be eaten raw with milk and honey.

Granola I

5 cups oat flakes or rye flakes
1/2 cup sesame seeds
1/4 cup honey
2 cups raisins

1 cup sunflower seeds
1/2 cup oil
5 cups wheat flakes or more oat
   flakes

Mix the oat or rye flakes, seeds, oil, and honey. Spread the mixture thinly on a cookie sheet. Roast 2 to 5 minutes in a 400° oven until light brown. Watch very closely; the flakes brown quickly. Remove the roasted flakes from the oven and mix quickly with the untoasted flakes and raisins to prevent the hot mixture from sticking together in lumps. Cool completely. Store in covered containers.

Granola II

1 pound rolled oats
4 ounces sesame seeds
4 ounces wheat germ
1/2 cup honey

4 ounces almonds, pecans or walnuts
4 ounces sunflower seeds
1/4 cup oil
4-6 ounces coconut or raisins (optional)

This recipe is included to offer a variation in measurement technique (ounces instead of cups). Prepare as Granola I.

Hotstuff for Chilly Mornings

1 cup oatmeal or whole wheat cereal
   (Wheatena, bulgar)

1 cup water or lowfat or skim milk
Cinnamon

Bring water to a boil. (Heat milk but do not boil.) Add cereal and simmer 5 minutes, stirring frequently. Add garnish and serve. Suggested garnishes: raisins or other dried fruit, cooked or fresh apples, berries, peaches, chopped nuts, coconut, or banana slices.

Sunny Morning Sundae

1 cup lowfat yogurt or lowfat milk
1/2 cup sliced fresh or cooked fruit
   (apples, pears, bananas, peaches,
   berries)

1/2 cup toasted wheat germ or uncooked oatmeal
Sunflower seeds or chopped nuts

Combine or layer in parfait dish, all ingredients and eat.

PANCAKES

Use buckwheat pancake mix, or mix your own, and help children measure oil and milk, and beat eggs. Let each child have a chance to ladle out his own portion and cook it to his taste. Children's initials or simple animal designs may be made by pouring batter into desired shapes.

Vocabulary: Skillet, sizzle, bubbles, taste, frying pan, batter, stir, syrup, hot, spatula, beat, temperature, pancake turner, turn sides.

If you like to mix your own batter, the following recipe may be used:

Beat well:	2 eggs
Beat in:	1 1/2 cups lowfat milk, 1 teaspoon honey or molasses, 3 tablespoons oil
Then beat in:	1 1/2 cups buckwheat or whole wheat flour; 1/4 teaspoon salt; 2 teaspoons baking powder
Optional:	1 grated apple and 1 teaspoon cinnamon 1 cup chopped nuts or sunflower seeds 1/2 cup wheat berry or alfalfa sprouts 1 cup fresh berries, 2 carrots, grated
Top with:	applesauce and cinnamon or: strawberries and lowfat yogurt or: 2 ripe mashed bananas, 1 tablespoon lemon juice 1/4 teaspoon cinnamon, 2 tablespoons honey, combined over low heat or: applebutter or: 1/2 cup orange juice, 1 tablespoon cornstarch, combined over low heat. Cook until thickened, then add 1/2 cup lowfat yogurt.

Cottage Cheese Pancakes

6 eggs, separated	2 cups lowfat cottage cheese
2/3 cup whole wheat flour	1/2 teaspoon salt
1 tablespoon sugar	1/8 teaspoon cream of tartar
Dash of cinnamon or	Oil or butter for frying
1 tablespoon orange rind, grated	

Beat together the egg yolks, cottage cheese, flour, sugar, salt, and a sprinkle of cinnamon or grated orange rind. In another bowl beat the egg whites with the cream of tartar until they are stiff but not dry. Fold the beaten whites gently into the cheese mixture and drop the batter by large spoonfuls onto oiled griddle or skillet. Choose topping from above, or delicious plain. Serves 6.

Dips, Spreads and Sandwich Fillings

Buttermilk Dip

1/2 cup rinsed or dry lowfat cottage cheese
4 cups (1 pound) shredded cheddar cheese

1/2 teaspoon nutmeg
2 cups buttermilk
1 clove crushed garlic
3 tablespoons cornstarch

Mix cheeses with cornstarch and nutmeg. Heat buttermilk with garlic over low heat until hot. Add cheese mixture, stirring constantly until cheeses are melted. Serve in a fondue dish with bite-sized bread pieces.

Cottage Cheese Spread

1 tablespoon grated onion
1 teaspoon chopped green pepper OR
  1 tablespoon chopped celery
1 teaspoon dill

1/4 cup chopped nuts
1/4 cup chopped dried fruit
2 teaspoons lemon juice

Combine 1/2 cup lowfat cottage cheese with either column of ingredients.

Guacamole

1 ripe avocado
1 small onion, finely chopped
1 teaspoon lemon juice
Salt and pepper

1 ripe tomato, finely chopped
1/4 cup boiled dressing or mayonnaise

Remove pit and peel. Mash pulp of avocado. Mix with other ingredients.

Hummus

1 cup cooked or canned garbanzo beans (also called chick peas)
1/4 cup tahini (sesame seed butter)
1 clove garlic, crushed
1 tablespoon salad oil

Juice of 1 1/2 lemons (about 1/2 cup)
2 sprigs parsley, chopped
Salt to taste

Buzz in blender until smooth or mash with fork. Add juice from beans if paste gets too thick.

Eggplant Spread I

Follow recipe for Hummus, substituting baked eggplant for garbanzo beans.

Eggplant Spread II

1 baked eggplant
2 large tomatoes peeled and chopped
1/2 cup finely chopped onions
1 clove crushed garlic

1/4 cup lemon juice
Salt and pepper to taste
1/4 cup chopped parsley
1/4 cup oil

Mix all ingredients together. Serve with whole wheat Pita bread.

Split Pea Spread

1 cup cooked green split peas
2 tablespoons salad dressing
3/4 cup toasted sunflower seeds
   (ground)

Salt to taste
Dash pepper
2 tablespoons lemon juice

Mash split peas and mix in other ingredients.

Split Pea—Parmesan Spread

1 cup cooked green split peas
2 tablespoons salad dressing
2 tablespoons parmesan cheese
2 tablespoons low fat cottage cheese

1/2 teaspoon basil
1/2 teaspoon salt
Dash of pepper

Mash split peas and mix in other ingredients.

Swiss Cheese Spread

1/2 cup grated Swiss cheese
1/2 cup low fat cottage cheese
1/4 cup chopped green pepper
1 tablespoon salad dressing

1/2 teaspoon dill weed
1/4 teaspoon mustard powder
Salt and pepper to taste

Mix the ingredients together and refrigerate until serving.

Yogurt Cream Cheese

Take about a half yard of clean cheesecloth and tie up the four corners to make a bag with an open top (or use a large coffee filter and cone shaped filter top coffee pot). Pour yogurt into filter, let stand over night. Pour homemade yogurt into the bag, tie a string around the top, and tie the string to the kitchen faucet. Let the liquid drain out of the yogurt into the sink for several hours or, in cool weather, overnight. Take the cheese out of the bag and season it with salt, finely chopped chives, and other herbs such as garlic, tarragon, parsley, and so forth. You can turn it into a dessert spread instead by using a little bit of salt, honey, and chopped nuts to taste.

Yogurt Dip

6 walnut halves
1 tablespoon oil
1/4 cup very finely diced peeled
   cucumber

1 clove garlic
1 cup low fat yogurt
1/2 teaspoon lemon juice
Whole grain crackers

Variations: add 1/2 teaspoon curry—use broccoli spears for dippers.

Place walnuts, garlic and oil in an electric blender and blend to a paste. Or use a mortar and pestle. Stir into the yogurt with cucumber and lemon juice. Chill and serve with crackers or raw vegetables as dippers. Serves 4.

Desserts

Apple Crisp

8-10 cooking apples or pears
3 cups raw rolled oat flakes
3/4 cup whole wheat flour
2/3 cup oil
2 teaspoons cinnamon
1/4 teaspoon salt

lemon juice
1/4 cup honey
1/2 cup orange juice
1 teaspoon allspice
chopped nuts (optional)
sunflower seeds (optional)

Pare and slice apples. Spread half of them into a 9" x 13" baking pan. Cover with lemon juice. Combine oat flakes, flour, oil, honey, spices, and nuts. Spread 1/2 the oat mixture onto apples in pan, and pat down. Cover with remaining apple slices, more lemon juice and remaining oat mix. Pour on 1/2 cup orange juice. Bake 40-45 minutes, uncovered, at 375°.

Baked Custard

2 cups milk plus 2 tablespoons
   powdered milk (or 3 tablespoons
   instant)
2 eggs, well beaten

2-3 tablespoons honey
1 teaspoon vanilla (or other flavoring—see below)

Beat the powdered milk into the whole milk OR you may use all powdered milk and water. Beat the eggs into the milk with a wire whisk; add the honey and vanilla. Pour the mixture into lightly oiled or buttered custard cups, or one baking dish. Place them in a pan of hot water filled to halfway up the sides of the cups or dish. Bake at 325°F. for about 50 minutes, until a knife inserted in the center comes out clean.

Variations:

Add 1 tablespoon carob powder to the basic recipe.

Add a few drops peppermint extract; omit vanilla.

Add a few drops almond extract; omit vanilla.

Stir in 1/4 to 1/2 cup lightly toasted unsweetened coconut. Add 1/2 cup chocolate or carob chips, too.

Buttermilk Coffee Cake

2 cups whole wheat flour
1/4 cup soy grits (optional)
1/4 teaspoon salt
2 teaspoon cinnamon
1 teaspoon baking soda
1 egg, beaten

1 teaspoon baking powder
1/2 cup raisins
3/4 cup honey
1/4 cup oil
1 cup buttermilk

Stir the raisins and the dry ingredients together. In a separate bowl beat the honey, oil, buttermilk, and egg together. Stir in the dry ingredients enough to blend them, but don't overblend. The littlest blending makes the tenderest cake. Pour into an oiled pan 11" x 7" and bake at 350°F. for 30-35 minutes.

Crunchy Banana Bread

3 ripe bananas
1 egg
1/3 cup honey
1/4 cup oil
1 teaspoon vanilla
1 1/2 cup whole wheat flour

1 teaspoon baking soda
1/2 teaspoon each salt, cinnamon,
ginger, cloves
1 cup sunflower seeds
1/3 cup chopped roasted peanuts
(optional)

In a large bowl mix together bananas, egg, honey, oil, and vanilla. Mix separately all other ingredients, then blend dry ingredients into liquid. Bake in an 8-inch-square pan for 1 hour at 350°F. The pan should be oiled and floured.

Frozen Fruit Yogurt

2 cups lowfat yogurt
1 small can frozen concentrated fruit
juice (orange or pineapple)

2 teaspoons vanilla

Combine all ingredients, mix well and place in refrigerator tray to freeze.

Fruit Fandango

10 crisp pears and/or apples
(Delicious are best), peeled

Cinnamon to taste
Strawberries, peaches (optional)

Cut up fruit into eighths. Simmer gently in sauce pan with enough water to keep from sticking (about 1/4 cup). Fruit should be firm, not mushy. Top with yogurt and serve hot or cold.

Gingerbread

2 1/4 cups whole wheat flour
1/4 teaspoon salt
1 teaspoon baking soda
2 teaspoons baking powder
1 cup unsulfured molasses

1 tablespoon freshly grated ginger
root
1 egg, beaten
1/4 cup oil
3/4 cup hot water

Stir the dry ingredients together (include the fresh ginger root here, too). Stir the remaining liquid ingredients together. They won't blend very well. Add the liquid to the dry mixture and blend with a few swift strokes. Immediately place the mixture in baking pan. Bake at 325°F for 30-35 minutes, until the cake tests done.

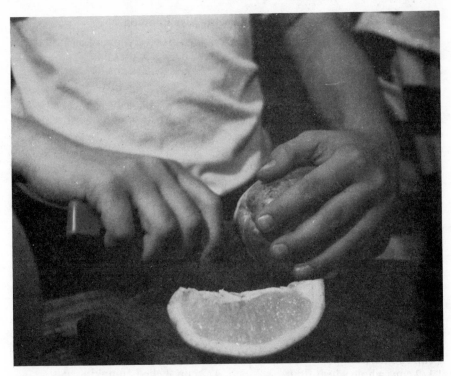

Molasses Oatmeal Cookies

1/3 cup oil
3 tablespoons honey
1 cup whole wheat flour
1 teaspoon cinnamon
1/8 teaspoon salt
1/2 teaspoon ground ginger
1/2 cup wheat germ

1/2 cup molasses
2 eggs, lightly beaten
1 teaspoon baking powder (optional)
1/2 teaspoon ground cloves
1/2 teaspoon allspice
2 cups rolled oats
1/2 cup raisins

Preheat the oven to 375°. Beat together the oil, molasses, honey and eggs. Sift together the whole wheat flour, baking powder, cinnamon, salt, cloves, ginger and allspice. Stir in the wheat germ, rolled oats and raisins. Add oil mixture to dry ingredients and mix well. Drop by teaspoonfuls onto oiled baking sheet and bake 8-10 minutes or until done. Cool on a rack. Serves about four dozen cookies.

Molasses Rice Pudding

1/3 cup brown rice
2 cups low fat milk
2 egg yolks
2 tablespoons molasses

3/4 cup chopped dates
1/4 teaspoon salt
2 egg whites
1 tablespoon sugar

Cook rice and milk in double boiler until tender (about 1 hour and 15 minutes). Pour over beaten egg yolks. Return to double boiler and add molasses, dates, salt. Cook two minutes. Beat egg whites stiff; add sugar gradually. Fold into rice mixture. Chill. Serves 4.

Old-Fashioned Creamy Rice Pudding

1 2/3 cups brown uncooked rice
1/2 teaspoon salt
2 teaspoons brown sugar (optional)
1 cup apples, chopped

1/4 teaspoon cinnamon or nutmeg
2 1/2 cups low fat milk
1/2 cup seedless raisins

Combine all ingredients in top of double boiler. Cook, covered, over boiling water until rice is tender and milk is almost absorbed, one hour, stirring frequently. Serve warm. Serves 6-8.

Pineapple Sherbet

3-4 tablespoons honey
3/4 cup unsweetened canned pineapple (or other fruit)
1 1/2 cups buttermilk

1 tablespoon lemon juice
rind of 1 lemon, grated
2 egg whites, beaten stiff

Blend honey and fruit. Add buttermilk, lemon juice and rind. Freeze until firm. Beat well and fold in egg whites. Freeze once again and serve. Serves 6.

Pumpkin Bread

1/2 cup honey
1/4 cup oil
2 eggs
1 cup cooked pumpkin
1 1/2 cups whole wheat flour
3/4 teaspoon salt

1/2 teaspoon baking powder
1 1/2 teaspoon cinnamon
1/2 teaspoon nutmeg
1/4 teaspoon cloves
1/2 cup shelled pumpkin seeds

Mix together honey and oil in bowl. Add eggs and beat well with egg beater. Add pumpkin and stir well. Sift dry ingredients together and add to pumpkin

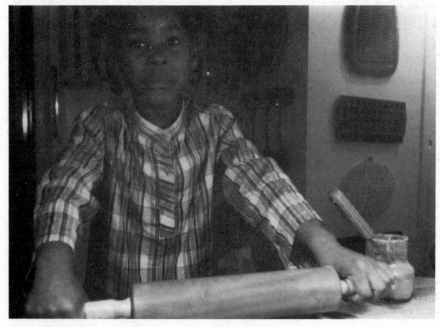

mixture, mixing well. Stir in pumpkin seeds. Pour into greased 5" x 9" loaf pan. Bake 1 hour at 325° or until cake tester comes out clean. Remove from oven. Turn out on wire rack and allow to cool before slicing.

Soybean Snacks

Put a cupful of rinsed soybeans into a bowl, cover them with water, and soak them in the refrigerator overnight. In the morning, drain the beans well and spread them out on a cookie sheet. Bake them in a 200°F. oven for 2 1/2 hours. Drizzle a teaspoonful of olive oil over the beans and stir them with a spoon until every bean looks oiled. Put them back into the oven for another half hour. As soon as you take them out, sprinkle them lightly with salt, if desired. When the beans are thoroughly cool, store them in a covered jar. Serve as you would salted nuts.

Sweet Potato Bread

2 large sweet potatoes
1 cup flour, whole wheat
1 teaspoon salt
2 tablespoons margarine, melted
2 eggs, lightly beaten
1 cup corn meal
1 teaspoon baking powder
2 tablespoons honey or molasses
1 1/4 cups warm lowfat milk

Parboil sweet potatoes for about 50 minutes or until just tender. Cool, peel and cut into 1/4" cubes. Sift together dry ingredients and place in a mixing bowl. Combine the honey, margarine, milk and eggs, and mix into the dry ingredients. Fold in the cubed sweet potatoes, pour batter into a well greased 8" x 8" x 2" baking dish and bake in a hot oven, 400°, for 1 hour. Serves 8-10.

Whole Wheat Pie Crust

2 cups whole wheat pastry flour
1/4 teaspoon salt
1/2 cup soft shortening, about 1/2 cup water

Stir the salt and whole wheat pastry flour together. Work the shortening in with a knife or pastry blender, but don't work it in too much. The pieces may be quite lumpy, but it will make a flakier crust. Add about 1/3 cup of water and move the crust mixture around so the water will soak in. Gather the dough gently and add more water if there is some flour that won't gather. Divide the dough in half, roll each half and fit into pie plates OR you may use half of the crust for an upper crust. If you are making an unbaked pie, bake the crust at 375°F. for 10 to 15 minutes. Prick the bottom with a fork so it will stay flat OR put about 1/4 cup of raw rice over the bottom to hold the crust down.

Yogurt Pie

1/2 pound lowfat cottage cheese
1 cup low fat yogurt
Fresh strawberries, raspberries,
    blueberries, or sliced bananas
1 tablespoon honey
1 teaspoon vanilla

Bake an 8-inch pie shell. Line the bottom with fresh strawberries, raspberries, blueberries or sliced bananas. Sprinkle with 1 tablespoon liquid honey. Whip together yogurt, cottage cheese, honey, and vanilla. Cover the fruit with the yogurt mixture and refrigerate for several hours before serving.

The Authors

Mary T. Goodwin, mother of three, has been the nutritionist for Montgomery County, Maryland, since 1969. She has long been concerned about promoting good nutrition based on natural foods. But more broadly, she believes that food is a uniquely effective means of getting children interested in ethnicity, their senses, math, older generations, and the community. At a time in which eating habits and personal beliefs are molded to a great extent by manufactured goods and advertising, Ms. Goodwin has served as a source of inspiration for progressive nutritionists and nutrition educators throughout the United States and Canada.

Mary Goodwin was born in Mabou, Nova Scotia, and was educated at St. Francis Xavier University (Antigonish, Nova Scotia), University of Toronto, and University of Maryland. In 1972 she was honored with an Achievement Award for her work in community nutrition by the National Association of Counties. She is author or co-author of several other books, including *Food: Where Nutrition, Politics and Culture Meet* and *Better Living Through Better Eating.*

Gerry Pollen earned her undergraduate degree at Barnard College, then went to Teachers College, Columbia University, where she received a Master's degree in education (with an emphasis on curriculum and teaching). She also has an Advanced Professional Certificate in early childhood education from the state of Maryland. Ms. Pollen has gained her insights into educating children through her eight years of experience at public and private schools in New York City and Long Island and seven years as a teacher and parent-trainer at the Beth-El Cooperative Pre-School in Bethesda, Maryland. In those situations she relished working with small children, who enthusiastically carried the nutrition message to their families. Her experience with her own two children also shows in this book. Gerry Pollen now works at the National Institutes of Health, where she spent almost two years as a program analyst for the Nutrition Coordinating Committee.

The Publisher

The Center for Science in the Public Interest is a non-profit, tax-exempt organization that is concerned about the effects of technology on society. Most of CSPI's work has focused on food, nutrition and health. CSPI has published numerous books, posters, and pamphlets for both teachers and the general public. In 1975, 1976 and 1977 CSPI sponsored National Food Day, and in 1979 it sponsored the Great American Nutrition Campaign, a coast-to-coast nutrition education campaign. In addition to educational activities, CSPI has been a Washington advocate for better food labeling, restrictions on the advertising on children's television shows, and bans on unsafe food additives.

For information about CSPI's publications and membership programs, please write to:

Center for Science in the Public Interest
1755 S St., NW
Washington, D.C. 20009